blood
pressure
all you need to know

Hugh Coni
Nicholas Coni

The ROYAL
SOCIETY *of*
MEDICINE
PRESS *Limited*

©2003 Royal Society of Medicine Press Ltd
1 Wimpole Street, London W1G 0AE, UK
207 E Westminster Road, Lake Forest, IL 60045, USA
www.rsmpress.co.uk

British Library Cataloguing in Publication Data
A catalogue record for this book is available from the British Library

ISBN 1-85315-536-5

Cartoons by GH Designs, UK
Typeset by Toby Matthews, London
Printed in Great Britain by Latimer Trend & Company Ltd, Plymouth

Contents

About the Authors

Hugh Coni MB BS BSc MRCGP trained at the Charing Cross and Westminster Medical School, London, and then attended the Portsmouth GP training scheme. He spent some time in Australia increasing his general medical experience prior to settling into general practice in Petersfield, Hampshire in 1999. Dr Coni is currently managing more than 270 people with hypertension, over 30 of whom choose to monitor their own blood pressure. Hypertension cases take up 13% of all his consultations and account for nearly 500 consultations per annum. Because of his interest and expertise, Dr Coni was invited to join the Information and Support Advisory Group to the Blood Pressure Association – the British 'forum for individuals whose lives are affected by blood pressure'. A period of serious illness at the outset of his career has given him a special insight into the experiences of his patients.

Nicholas Coni MA FRCP (London & Canada) qualified from Cambridge University and Westminster Medical School, and after various hospital posts was appointed to the consultant staff of Addenbrooke's Hospital, Cambridge in 1970. After serving on the Health Authority, he became clinical director of the Department of Medicine for the Elderly. Dr Coni has authored many papers in medical journals and chapters of books on medical subjects. He also taught the medical students of Cambridge University. Now retired, he participates in the activities of the University of the Third Age in Cambridge (of which he was co-founder) and takes a keen interest in the management of his own hypertension.

Foreword

Hypertension has been one of the success stories of modern medicine, up to a point – it is easy to diagnose (in most patients) and relatively easy to treat (in most patients). When writing a prescription for hypertension, we have more classes of drugs to choose from than when prescribing for any other common condition. Most of these drug classes have been shown as effective not only in reducing blood pressure, but also in preventing the long-term complications of hypertension, namely heart attacks and strokes. Yet most patients either do not receive the drugs that they need or have not been convinced that daily consumption of medicines for an asymptomatic condition is, as CS Lewis might have said, 'the pain now that pays for the pleasure of avoiding strokes later'. Although hypertension is listed by the World Health Organization as the third most important cause of morbidity in the western world (after smoking and alcohol), there are only a handful of specialists in the UK. We therefore need help to spread information about the nature and importance of hypertension, and so the target audience of this book is particularly appropriate. Until a few years ago, the specialists, lacking evidence to the contrary, took the somewhat condescending view that high blood pressure in older people was a good thing, helping to push blood down the hardening arteries. Now we know, as the Conis illustrate well, that the contrary is true. Older people stand to gain the most from having their blood pressure lowered – simply because they are the most at risk if it is not.

Our confidence in our understanding of what hypertension is and what causes it is on shakier ground than our conviction about the merits of treatment. We understand well enough how blood pressure is controlled in healthy subjects; and at a superficial level we can divide hypertension into two types depending on the age of presentation (as in diabetes). Type 1, in younger patients, is associated with raised levels of the kidney hormone renin and responds well to drugs that suppress the renin system, eg ACE inhibitors and beta-blockers. Type 2, in older patients, is associated with suppressed levels of renin and responds best to drugs which eliminate salt and elevate renin, eg calcium channel blockers and diuretics. The serendipitous sequence of these drugs' initials has let us enunciate an ABCD of hypertension – a rule which at once explains the condition and recommends appropriate treatment.

But peer below the surface, and our understanding of hypertension becomes vague – appropriate, perhaps, for a condition which we diagnose with a stethoscope applied to a large artery in the arm, but whose origins lie in the almost invisible arterial branches at the end of the arterial tree. We live in an era when true understanding of a disease demands not only detailed *dramatis personae*, goodies and baddies, in the form of multiple molecular sequences, but also an entire script for how these interact scene by scene. Not so long ago, professors argued for their favourite candidate gene as the single cause of hypertension – as likely to be resolved as the number of angels dancing on a pin. It took genetic studies of the well-recognized inherited contribution to hypertension to show that no single gene is responsible and that the number of genes involved is probably as large as that of the angels. Progress is being made in this research, but as the rate of progress slows, our confidence that genetics will provide the main answers to hypertension is ebbing away. This book explores some of the alternatives, including the controversial idea that we can blame our cardiovascular risk on our mothers' habits during pregnancy.

Whether the causes of hypertension will be found in our parents or our stars, books like this help to ensure that the consequences of hypertension will be strongly influenced by ourselves. Further knowledge of the causes of hypertension might satisfy intellectual curiosity and may eventually lead to yet more choice of treatments; but all patients can now have knowledge of the consequences and how to prevent them. The Conis draw on their rich and varied experience of hypertension in everyday practice to impart this knowledge in an intelligent and intelligible fashion. After all, 'the patient with knowledge is the patient in control'.

Morris J Brown
MA, MSc, MD, FRCP, FMedSci
Member of the Executive Committee of the British Hypertension Society; Professor of Clinical Pharmacology, University of Cambridge, Cambridge, UK; Consultant Physician, Addenbrooke's Hospital, Cambridge, UK

Preface

Diseases are important for many reasons: because they are common, because they can be fatal, because they cause a great deal of disability, because they cause considerable suffering or because of their great cost to society. Hypertension fulfils all these criteria.

More and more people develop hypertension as they grow older and it is unbelievably prevalent among middle-aged and elderly people in the developed world. It probably affects over half the population aged over 65 years of industrialized countries and is mankind's most common chronic disease. Hypertension is associated with a very high mortality, especially from related coronary artery disease and stroke. Survivors of stroke comprise approximately 25% of severely disabled people living within the community. Few disorders can therefore have such a legitimate claim to be one of the greatest afflictions of our time.

Hypertension is almost always without symptoms. When we say 'I suffer from hypertension', we do not mean we are really 'suffering' in the accepted sense of the word. What we actually mean is that a doctor, or perhaps a life insurance company, has strongly hinted that they do not think we are going to live as long as we had hoped. Paradoxically, hypertension causes headache – but only in those who have been told they have hypertension!

This is what has made hypertension such an unfashionable disease. Not only is it very unglamorous, conjuring up cartoon images of portly, middle-aged, puce-faced business men, but even those afflicted do not really want to know about it. Who wishes to be constantly reminded of their own mortality? And as for doctors – a great deal of their job satisfaction comes from making people feel better, but you cannot make a symptom-free individual feel better with pills, although you can certainly make them feel worse.

Hypertension is therefore not always treated or monitored in the most appropriate ways, either by hospital specialists, GPs or those who have the condition. A visit to the out-patient clinic at the hospital is likely to be associated with:

- ❖ the stress of getting time off work
- ❖ a difficult journey to the hospital
- ❖ problems parking the car

❖ problems finding the right clinic

❖ being kept waiting before a brief consultation with a stranger.

Consequently, hypertension is mainly dealt with by GPs – the surgery may be closer, the parking easier and the nurse less intimidating, but visits are still likely to be very infrequent. No wonder that in the surgery, doctors are inclined to be satisfied with blood pressure levels that may be higher than are desirable, and simply hope that the rest of the time, the readings would be lower.

The best hope for all the hundreds of thousands, probably millions, of people with hypertension is to cultivate an informed interest in the subject, just like many diabetics take a keen interest in diabetes. They need to take charge of their own blood pressure control, loosely under the supervision of the GP or the specialist, to take their own readings which they share with their medical adviser, to adopt sensible lifestyle changes and to discuss their medication. They need to become what the Department of Health has called 'expert patients' – an idea borrowed from the University of Stanford, California. This book will try to educate those affected and their families to enable them to do so. The authors are a GP who undertakes the supervision of most of the hypertensive patients in his practice and a recently retired hospital physician who takes regular medication for high blood pressure.

During the 1990s, a new buzz-word (or buzz-phrase) infiltrated medi-speak: it was 'evidence-based medicine' (EBM). Medicine has, in fact, been evidence-based ever since Sir Austin Bradford Hill devised the trials which were to provide statistical proof of the effectiveness of certain drugs against tuberculosis in the late 1940s and early 1950s – EBM was not exactly a new idea! Most of the information in this book is evidence-based, and so is the general concept that the 'expert patient' enjoys improved healthcare outcomes. However, we have to acknowledge that the core themes of this book (dissemination of information to the public and self-measurement of blood pressure) are only now beginning to enjoy an evidence base. Nevertheless one can die of a heart attack or a stroke while waiting for the evidence to become rock-solid, and there are a few ideas which are so intuitively right, so devoid of adverse effects, and so inexpensive, that it does seem reasonable to try them while waiting for the evidence to accumulate.

We have tried to set out as much information on the subject as possible, in what we hope is a reasonably 'jargon-free' manner. Some of the medical terminology is unavoidable and we have tried to provide explanations where necessary. We have devoted the majority of the book to high blood pressure but have included information on normal blood pressure and also low blood pressure. If anyone picks up this book and finds the subject becomes more interesting than they anticipated, writing it will have been worth while.

Nurses, who are undertaking an increasing proportion of the detection and supervision of hypertensive subjects in primary care, will also find the book informative, and we believe that medical students and pharmacists will find it a useful handbook.

Abbreviations

ACE	angiotensin-converting enzyme
ADH	antidiuretic hormone
AE	adverse effects
ANS	autonomic nervous system
BP	blood pressure
CHD	coronary heart disease
CNS	central nervous system
CO	cardiac output
CVS	cardiovascular system
DBP	diastolic blood pressure
ECG	electrocardiogram
GP	general practitioner
HDL	high-density lipoprotein (cholesterol)
HRT	hormone replacement therapy
ISH	isolated systolic hypertension
JNC	Joint National Committee. Sixth report on hypertension (USA) 1997
LA	left atrium
LDL	low-density lipoprotein (cholesterol)
LV	left ventricle
LVH	left ventricular hypertrophy
MABP	mean arterial pressure
MI	myocardial infarction
NHS	National Health Service
PR	peripheral resistance
RA	right atrium
RAS	renin–angiotensin system
RV	right ventricle
SBP	systolic blood pressure
SBPM	self blood pressure measurement
SV	stroke volume

Chapter One

The circulation and the blood pressure

In order to understand the blood pressure, its disorders and their treatment, it is necessary to have some knowledge of the blood circulation. Here we describe something of the **anatomy** (structure) and **physiology** (function) of the heart and blood vessels and their contribution to the blood pressure. We also discuss what the blood pressure actually is and what sort of level can be described as 'normal'.

How does the heart pump blood around the body?

Before describing the various disorders of the blood pressure, it seems logical to start with a brief account of the blood circulation (Figure 1.1).

In the average adult, the circulatory system contains approximately five litres of blood (eight imperial pints), and this is the **circulating blood volume**. At rest, the heart will pump almost this amount of blood around the body each minute. At this rate, the heart will pump out 7200 litres of blood per day – weighing 100 times more than the average human body. The blood pumped by the heart takes 250 ml of oxygen each minute from the lungs to the body tissues, all of which are completely dependent on this supply of oxygen.

Assuming that a person is resting, the heart will beat approximately 70 times each minute (the **heart rate**), although the rate is variable and depends on many factors other than the level of

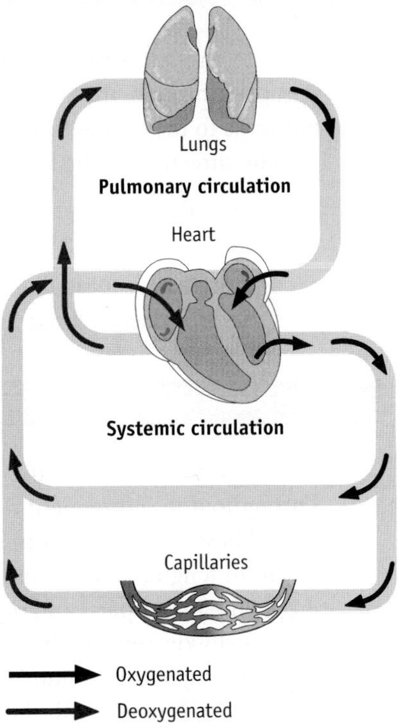

Lungs

Pulmonary circulation

Heart

Systemic circulation

Capillaries

Figure 1.1 The circulation of the blood. Diagrammatic representation of the heart, lungs and circulation.

⟶ Oxygenated
⟶ Deoxygenated

> The average human adult body contains about five litres pf blood

physical activity. Therefore, each heartbeat propels about 70 ml of blood from the left side of the heart into the **aorta**, the great arterial motorway where the journey around the circulation begins. The amount of blood pumped into the aorta during each heartbeat is known as the **stroke volume**.

Where CO is cardiac output, SV is stroke volume, and HR is heart rate, it is easy to see that:

$$CO = SV \times HR$$

In the example above, the **cardiac output** would be 4900 mL per minute.

As Figure 1.1 indicates, there are effectively two separate circulations each fed by their own pump. Each pump corresponds to one side of the heart and has two chambers:

- ❖ the **atria** or receiving chambers
- ❖ the highly muscular **ventricles** or ejecting chambers.

> The main artery that takes blood to the organs is called the aorta; the main veins that transport blood back to the heart are the superior and inferior vena cava

The right ventricle sends blood into the pulmonary circulation via the pulmonary arteries. These vessels take the blood to the lungs where it releases carbon dioxide and soaks up oxygen. The blood returns through the pulmonary veins to the left atrium, flows through a valve to the left ventricle and is then pumped through the aorta to the arteries. After delivering oxygen and other nutrients to the tissues, blood returns through the veins to the right atrium.

The direction of the bloodstream through the heart is secured by valves:

- ❖ One valve is situated between each atrium and ventricle to prevent the ventricle forcing blood backwards into the atrium.
- ❖ One valve is located at the outlet of each ventricle, so as the heart relaxes between beats, it does not refill with the blood it has just ejected.

The blood vessels

The aorta loops over in the chest in the shape of a question mark (Figure 1.2). Throughout its subsequent descent into the abdomen, numerous arteries branch off it. These arteries differ in size; if the aorta, measuring 2–3 cm in diameter and 50 cm in length, is the 'motorway', the large arteries are the 'trunk roads' which supply the major parts and organs of the body. On arrival at their destinations, the arteries divide repeatedly into smaller arteries and then into **arterioles**, which have a diameter of around 70 millionths of a metre (μm). Arterioles are therefore too small to be seen with the naked eye. The arterioles branch yet again to form

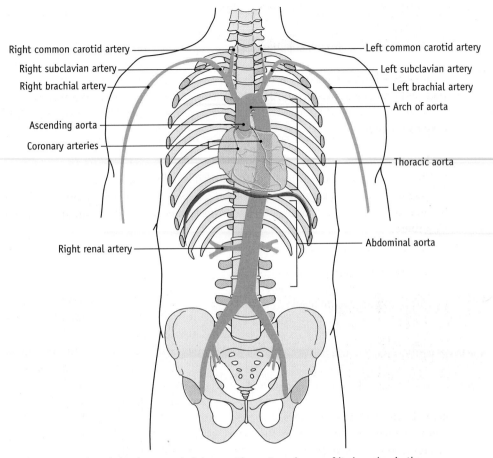

Right common carotid artery — — Left common carotid artery

Right subclavian artery — — Left subclavian artery

Right brachial artery — — Left brachial artery

— Arch of aorta

Ascending aorta —

Coronary arteries —

— Thoracic aorta

Right renal artery — — Abdominal aorta

Figure 1.2 Arteries of the thorax and abdomen. The aorta and some of its branches in the thorax and abdomen.

the **capillaries** (10 μm or less in diameter). Capillaries are so narrow that red blood cells, which are 7 or 8 μm wide, are only just able to pass along them.

The capillaries are the vessels that are in the most intimate contact with body cells and the fluid which bathes them, and it is here that the vital functions of the microcirculation take place. To pursue the motorway analogy, these are the little pedestrian precincts in the centre of the city, where the miniscule day to day transactions involving the exchange of life's necessities are carried out.

> The smallest blood vessels, the capillaries, are so narrow that red blood cells can only just flow though them

Collectively, all the capillaries are often referred to as the **capillary bed**. After the exchange of oxygen and nutrients for carbon dioxide and waste products has been completed, the blood needs to be returned to the heart so that it can:

3

❖ be sent to the lungs to dispose of the carbon dioxide which had accumulated in the tissues

❖ pick up new oxygen supplies.

Table 1.1: Vessels of the circulation

Type of vessel	Diameter (mm)	Number in parallel	Total area (cm²)
Aorta	25	1	2.5
Arteries	2	600	5
Arterioles	0.07	50 million	40
Capillaries	0.005–0.01	1000 million	1,700
Venules	0.03	100 million	375
Great veins	13	2	10

Table 1.2: Location of blood at any instant in a resting individual

Structure	% blood
Pulmonary circulation	12
Heart	6
Arteries + arterioles	11
Capillaries	5
Veins & venules	66

Therefore, capillaries reunite with each other to form **venules**, and these gradually join up to form the great veins which take blood to the right atrium.

It has been estimated that the body of an adult may contain 60,000 miles of blood vessels. An approximate idea of the relative scale of the vessels of the circulation is given in Table 1.1, and the amount of blood present in the various parts of the circulation at any given moment is detailed in Table 1.2.

Where does all the blood go to?

Table 1.3: Distribution of blood flow at rest

Organ	Blood flow (litres per min)
Brain	0.75
Heart muscle	0.25
Other muscles	1.2
Skin	0.5
Kidneys	1.1
Gut	1.4

The supply of blood to a region or organ is called the **perfusion** of that region or organ. Table 1.3 shows how much of the output from the heart is allocated to the perfusion of different organs in the resting state. The distribution of the blood can be adjusted to meet special requirements, such as during exercise or a cold environment (see Chapter 2, p18).

What makes the blood return to the heart?

The heart muscle pumps the blood out through the 'arterial tree' to the tissues, but the force of its contractions is progressively weakened as the blood moves down the arterioles and into the capillary bed. By the time the blood has reached the venules, the pumping force from the heart is hardly felt. There are three main forces that help the venous circulation:

❖ gravity – in the case of the head and neck, and the arms when elevated

❖ the negative pressure generated within the thorax every time we inhale, which sucks the blood into the heart

❖ the pumping action of the leg muscles – the muscles squeeze the leg veins and the blood within the veins can only proceed in an upwards direction due to a system of internal valves.

Guardsmen and soldiers are liable to faint when they stand motionless because blood tends to pool in the lower extremities, starving the heart and therefore the brain of blood and oxygen. Attempting to make imperceptible leg movements may prevent the soldier from actually passing out.

Structure of blood vessels

The different types of blood vessel have several striking differences in their structure (Figure 1.3). This is because they have very different functions. Both arteries and veins consist of:

❖ two layers of muscle lined on the inside by a single layer of smooth **endothelial cells**

❖ variable quantities of collagen, a relatively rigid protein

❖ variable quantities of elastin, a highly stretchable protein.

There is more collagen in the walls of the arteries and arterioles and more elastin in the walls of veins and venules. Capillaries lack the layers of muscle and are constructed only of endothelium. Fluid, rich in essential nutrients and the waste products of metabolism, can pass to-and-fro through the capillary walls.

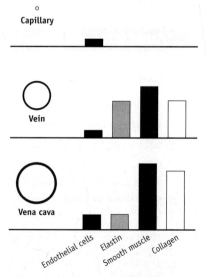

Figure 1.3 Blood vessel walls. The structure of the different blood vessel walls varies in thickness and composition.

The walls of the arteries contain more muscle than the veins – after trauma, contraction of this muscle helps to staunch bleeding

The arteries are more muscular and much thicker-walled than the veins. This is important for the body to achieve damage limitation following trauma. Being directly downstream of the heart, arterial bleeding is often torrential. Muscular contraction leading to constriction of the artery (**vasoconstriction**) is the first line of defence and reduces the flow before the blood-clotting mechanism has time to act. Vasoconstriction is more effective in younger subjects as older people have more collagen in their arterial walls, which renders them stiffer and less able to constrict.

What happens between heartbeats?

The contraction of the ventricles is called **systole** and the interval between contractions when the ventricles are refilling with blood is called **diastole**. During

Systole is the contraction of the heart and diastole is the interval between heartbeats

systole, the aorta and the large arteries do stretch, but only to a limited extent. This requires a considerable amount of energy, which is stored in the vessel walls. During diastole, this energy is released in the form of elastic recoil. This squeezing effect helps to maintain the blood pressure and the flow of blood through the capillaries.

What is the peripheral resistance?

Arterioles are muscular and many times more numerous than the arteries. However, their number is low compared to that of the capillaries and venules (Table 1.1). When the muscle contracts, the arteriole constricts; when this process is occurring simultaneously in a large proportion of the arterioles, their total cross section becomes greatly reduced and the resistance to the forward flow of blood is increased. For this reason, the arterioles are sometimes classified as **resistance vessels**.

When the muscle in the arteriole wall relaxes, the vessel dilates (**vasodilatation**). Constriction or dilatation of the arterioles supplying a particular

Table 1.4: How different vessels contribute to the peripheral resistance

Blood vessels	% of peripheral resistance
Arterioles	40
Arteries	25
Capillaries	20
Venous system	15

tissue will determine what proportion of the cardiac output reaches that tissue's capillaries. The total of all the resistances of the arterioles supplying the **systemic circulation** (as opposed to pulmonary circulation) is the major constituent of the total **peripheral resistance** (Table 1.4). Peripheral resistance is the resistance to the passage of blood through the systemic circulation.

What about the resistance in the veins and venules?

The veins and venules contain a great deal of elastin in their comparatively thin walls, which makes them very stretchy, or **compliant**. At any given moment, they contain a very high proportion of the total circulating blood volume. The veins and venules are capable of holding large, variable quantities of blood without the pressure within them fluctuating dramatically. They are therefore often referred to as **capacitance vessels**.

> The veins and venules are stretchy due to the protein elastin in their walls – these vessels can hold very variable quantities of blood

What has all this to do with the blood pressure?

When we talk about the blood pressure (BP), we are speaking of:

❖ the pressure in the systemic rather than the pulmonary circulation

❖ the measurable pressure within the large arteries and not in the veins

❖ the pressure in a large, readily accessible artery in the arm – although this may seem quite far from the heart, the pressure has not yet decreased significantly. By the time blood reaches the capillaries, the pressure is very much lower.

When giving a BP reading, two figures are always given – the systolic (SBP) and the diastolic (DBP). The reading is therefore the

> Normally, blood pressure is measured in the brachial artery in the arm

pressures during these two phases of the heart's action. The difference between the SBP and the DBP is the **pulse pressure** and the **mean arterial blood pressure** (MABP) is taken to be the DBP plus one-third of the pulse pressure.

The BP depends upon three factors:

❖ the blood volume (see Chapter 2, p15)

❖ the cardiac output (CO)

❖ the peripheral resistance (PR).

For any given blood volume, the latter two are expressed by the mathematical formula:

$$MABP = CO \times PR$$

Put very simply:

❖ the higher the cardiac output (hence heart rate and stroke volume) and peripheral resistance, the higher the BP

❖ the lower the cardiac output and peripheral resistance, the lower the BP.

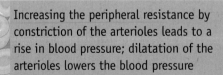

Increasing the peripheral resistance by constriction of the arterioles leads to a rise in blood pressure; dilatation of the arterioles lowers the blood pressure

The way the BP is usually expressed looks like a fraction, but is really just the SBP above the line and the DBP below the line.

What is the 'normal' BP?

There is really no such thing as a 'normal' BP – it varies enormously, not just between individuals, but in the same individual from time to time. The figure that is generally quoted to medical students as being 'normal' is 120/80 mmHg (measured in mm of mercury).

For those concerned for the welfare of their domestic pets, it may be added that measuring the BP in other animals is, for obvious reasons, a much less

Table 1.5: 'Normal' blood pressure levels in animals

Animal	'Normal' BP (mmHg)	Additional information
Horse	112/77	High BP may cause nosebleeds
Cattle	100–140/50–85	
Dog	112–148/56–87	Hypertension causes heart failure, stroke or kidney failure
Cat	104–171/73–123	
Mouse	81	(MABP)
Rat	130/91	Hypertension causes stroke
Frog	30/20	
Salmon	30/22	
Octopus	44/22	
Lobster	13/1	At rest
	27/13	When active
Giraffe	280/80	

routine part of a medical examination than it is in humans. 'Normal' levels in other species are less well documented. Table 1.5 shows some figures for other animals.

Investigations have found that continuous emotional arousal of a solitary animal, ie lone family pet, will eventually lead to a measure of chronic hypertension.

Age and the blood pressure

Older people have more collagen in their arterial walls than younger people. This makes the arteries stiffer and less elastic. The arteries

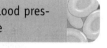

In the developed world, blood pressure tends to rise with age

of a 70-year-old are said to be only 50% as compliant ('stretchy') as those of a young adult. A decrease in arterial distensibility ('elasticity') causes the SBP to rise. In the developed world it is exceedingly common to find that the BP, especially the SBP, rises with age (Table 1.6).

The figures in Table 1.6 are often quoted, but they are also hotly disputed. It all depends on what you mean by 'normal' – the word is used in two quite different senses:

❖ It can be taken to mean what is common in the UK (or France or the USA or wherever the speaker happens to reside).

Table 1.6: 'Normal' BPs at different ages

Age (years)	Blood pressure (mmHg)
5–10	90/60
13–18	105/65
22–25	120/80
35	130/85
45	140/90
55	145/95
65	150/95
75	150/100

❖ It can be used to denote someone who is healthy and free from disease.

Table 1.6 is only valid in the former sense. But, using the latter definition of normality, the figures from age 35 onwards are distinctly worrying.

Other factors affecting the BP

The cardiac output influences the BP and the stroke volume influences the cardiac output. An increase in the heart rate is the main factor in the rise in cardiac output that occurs during exercise (see Chapter 2, p17). Many day-to-day events influence the BP on a transient basis (see Chapter 7, p61).

There are some long-term situations in which the stroke volume is elevated, resulting in a fall in the DBP and possibly a slight rise in the SBP so that the pulse pressure is larger. These include:

❖ pregnancy

❖ very slow pulse (highly trained athletes or heart block, which is when conduction of the heartbeat from its natural pacemaker has been interrupted)

❖ severe anaemia

❖ high fever

❖ disease of the aortic valve (between the left ventricle and the aorta).

Conclusion

Much of the information in this chapter will initially seem to have little relevance to most of the readers of this book, many of whom will have hypertension. But one of the core themes of the book is that hypertension is like diabetes: if you have the condition, you are well advised to study it, to become absorbed in it, to become an authority on it. An understanding of the physiology of the BP is a prerequisite to understanding the control of the BP and the mechanisms by which the various drugs exert their beneficial (and adverse) effects.

Summary points

❖ We have described the circulation of the blood: the blood pressure measured is the pressure prevailing in the arteries and is usually measured in the main artery in the arm.

❖ The pressure during cardiac contractions (SBP) is higher than that during the phase of relaxation (DBP); these two figures are quoted in a blood pressure reading.

❖ With any given blood volume, the mean arterial blood pressure is the product of the stroke volume and the peripheral resistance.

❖ The muscular arterioles (the 'resistance vessels') are responsible for the peripheral resistance.

❖ The frequently quoted level for a 'normal' blood pressure is 120/80 mmHg, but higher levels are extremely prevalent, especially in older people.

❖ People who have hypertension are advised to learn about the condition and understand the physiology and management of this serious disorder.

Chapter Two

How does the body control blood pressure?

Our bodies have numerous inbuilt mechanisms whereby many biological measurements are maintained at an almost constant level. The **autonomic nervous system** (ANS) is the part of the nervous system that performs its functions without our conscious control. The ANS has a crucial role in the control of the blood pressure, and the kidneys also have an important role.

The interior of the body can be described in terms of a number of measurable chemical and physical parameters:

❖ The chemical parameters are the quantity and composition of fluid in the cells, tissue spaces and circulation. This includes the acidity or alkalinity of fluids such as plasma, and the concentrations of many constituents, such as sodium ions, potassium ions, chloride ions, sugar and various waste products.

❖ The physical parameters are primarily the body temperature and the pressure within the various fluid compartments.

Although these parameters can vary, wide fluctuations are extremely danger-ous. Mammals have developed some highly sophisticated systems to reduce the limits within which they vary and to maintain the constancy of what the French physiologist Claude Bernard (1813–1878) termed the milieu intérieure. This ability to pre-serve the internal environment even

> The mechanism of maintaining a con-stant internal environment within the body is called 'homeostasis'

in the face of a hostile external environment is known as **homeostasis**. The organs chiefly responsible for homeostatic mechanisms are the kidneys and the autonomic nervous system.

Blood pressure (BP) depends on the cardiac output and the peripheral resist-ance (Chapter 1, p8). The main constituent of the peripheral resistance is the network of arterioles, whose diameter is controlled by muscle (p6).

❖ The ANS is involved in the contraction of **smooth muscle**. The smooth muscle in the walls of the arterioles is similar to that in the walls of the intestines and other internal tubular structures. It is not subject to conscious control, but receives signals via the ANS that you are unaware of sending. The

> The autonomic nervous system controls the smooth muscle of the arterioles

main functions of the ANS are controlling smooth muscle and the secretions of certain glands.

❖ The central nervous system (CNS) also controls muscles. However, these muscles are under voluntary control, eg the biceps. Messages are sent through the CNS from the brain and the muscle will contract when you want.

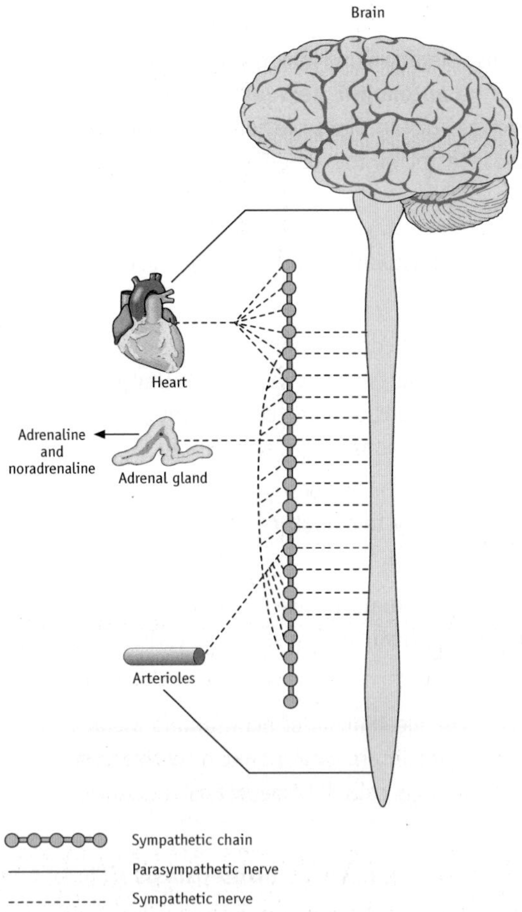

Most of the time, voluntary muscles contract when you want them to. You tell your right hand to pick the book up from the table, not which muscles should contract, and in what order they should do so. Occasionally a muscle will contract without receiving a signal from the brain; for example, when the doctor taps a knee tendon with a hammer, or when you touch something very hot. These muscle contractions are called **reflex actions**. During a reflex action the brain is bypassed – the circuit the message takes only involves the spinal cord and the incoming and outgoing nerves. The ANS does receive messages from certain parts of the brain but its main actions are triggered by reflexes.

The ANS consists of two separate divisions, which often have opposing effects – the **sympathetic** and the **parasympathetic** systems (Figure 2.1).

❖ Nerve fibres from the sympathetic division emerge from the CNS throughout the thoracic and lumbar (central) parts of the spinal cord.

Brain

Heart

Adrenaline and noradrenaline

Adrenal gland

Arterioles

○–○–○–○–○ Sympathetic chain

———— Parasympathetic nerve

– – – – – – Sympathetic nerve

Figure 2.1 The autonomic nervous system.
Diagrammatic representation of the two divisions of the autonomic nervous system and how they help control the blood pressure. (Connections of the ANS to numerous other organs are not shown.)

❖ Nerves from the parasympathetic division emerge from the brain stem and from the sacral (lowest) part of the spinal cord.

The chemicals which enable the nervous system to function are known as **neurotransmitters**.

> The autonomic nervous system is made up of two separate divisions – the sympathetic and parasympathetic systems

What do neurotransmitters do?

Each nerve cell (Figure 2.2), or **neurone**, consists of:

❖ a cell body which both receives and generates nervous impulses

❖ a long fibre (axon) which transmits the impulses.

At the end of each nerve fibre there is a tiny gap or cleft. On the other side of the cleft, there is either another nerve cell ready to receive and pass on the impulse, or there is an **effector cell**, eg a muscle or glandular cell waiting to spring into action on receiving the impulse. The cleft between two neurones is known as a **synapse** and measures 20 or 30 millionths of a millimetre. The cleft between a neurone and an effector cell is three or four times as wide as a synapse. For comparison, a red blood cell measures about 8 thousandths of a millimetre across, ie over 3000 times wider than a synapse.

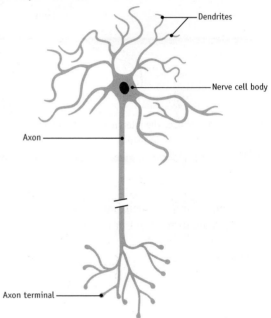

Figure 2.2 A nerve cell. Diagrammatic representation of a nerve cell; proportions here are misleading as the axon may be up to 10,000 times longer than the cell body is wide.

When the nerve impulse arrives at a cleft, a minute quantity of a neurotransmitter is released and diffuses across the gap (Figure 2.3). The neurotransmitter binds with receptors and triggers either an impulse in the next neurone or specific activity in an effector cell. Neurotransmitters involved in controlling blood pressure are:

> Neurotransmitters transmit nervous impulses from one nerve cell, across a cleft, to another nerve cell or effector cell

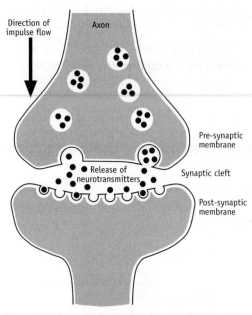

Figure 2.3 A synapse. The release and diffusion of neurotransmitter across a synaptic cleft – the junction between two nerve cells.

❖ **adrenaline**

❖ **noradrenaline**

❖ **acetylcholine.**

The effector cells we are mainly concerned with are the smooth muscle cells of the blood vessels. These cells receive impulses from sympathetic fibres, mostly transmitted by noradrenaline. Noradrenaline generally causes vasoconstriction, particularly in the arterioles of the skin, kidney and gut, thus elevating the peripheral resistance. The receptors in these arterioles are known as alpha adrenergic receptors.

The sympathetic nervous system also activates the adrenal gland to produce adrenaline. Because different types of receptor predominate in different sites, adrenaline and noradrenaline produce the same effects in some tissues and different effects in others:

> The actions of adrenaline are said to prepare us for 'fight or flight'

❖ in the skin, kidney and gut, adrenaline and noradrenaline cause arterioles to vasoconstrict

❖ adrenaline and noradrenaline cause the arterioles of the heart muscle to dilate and adrenaline also dilates arterioles in skeletal muscle.

Effects of the ANS on the heart

The sympathetic nerve supply and adrenaline exert similar effects on the heart muscle:

❖ they increase the heart rate

❖ they increase the force of the heart's contractions.

> Both adrenaline and the sympathetic nervous system increase the heart rate and the force of each contraction of the heart muscle

Both of the above effects augment the cardiac output as a result of the stimulation of the **beta adrenergic receptors** (see 'beta-blockers' in Chapter 10, p89).

The role of the kidneys

The kidneys respond to chemicals, some of which are instrumental in maintaining the BP. The most important of these chemicals is **antidiuretic hormone** (ADH). Antidiuretic hormone reduces the output of urine. It is secreted by the pituitary gland in response to the blood plasma becoming more concentrated, eg when an organism becomes dehydrated. The secretion of ADH is therefore an important homeostatic mechanism because it conserves the blood volume. A sudden drop in blood volume (eg as occurs in haemorrhage) also causes the release of ADH. It also has important properties as a potent vasoconstrictor, thereby maintaining the BP.

The other important contribution made by the kidneys to BP control is the **renin–angiotensin** system. The protein **angiotensinogen**, which is synthesized in the liver, is split by the enzyme **renin**, which is produced in the kidney, to yield **angiotensin I** (Figure 2.4). This is altered by **angiotensin-converting enzyme**

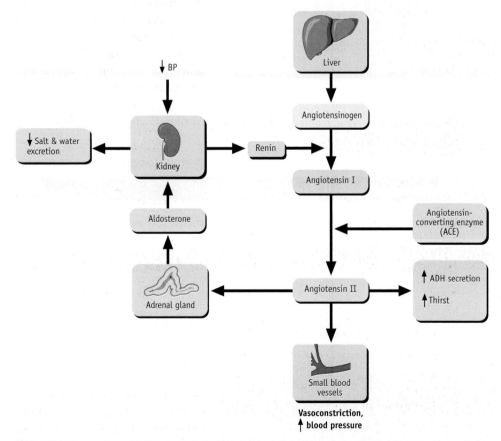

Figure 2.4 The renin–angiotensin system. The renin–angiotensin system and its effects on some of the organs of the body. ADH, antidiuretic hormone.

> Angiotensin-converting enzyme leads to the production of angiotensin II – an important vasoconstrictor

to make **angiotensin II**, which has an analogous effect to antidiuretic hormone on the conservation of fluid. Angiotensin II is also a potent vasoconstrictor and hence elevates the peripheral resistance. The rate of renin release from the kidney rises if the BP falls.

What is autoregulation?

One of the factors determining the level of blood flow to the various vital organs is the **perfusion pressure**. There is a homeostatic mechanism at work whereby even if the perfusion pressure changes considerably, the blood flow is kept fairly constant. This is called **autoregulation**, but just how it works remains uncertain.

> Blood flow to vital organs is kept fairly constant by 'autoregulation' although it is not fully understood how this process actually works

Autoregulation is particularly important in preserving blood flow to the brain and is much less effective in people who have a raised BP, so a drop in BP is likely to affect the function of the brain. One of the problems of low blood pressure, when the limits of autoregulation are exceeded, is the distress and danger that can result when there is a reduced blood supply to the brain (see Chapter 12, p113).

How do environmental stresses affect the BP?

Various challenges can affect the circulation in such a way as to present a threat to the constancy of the BP.

Effect of gravity

One might anticipate that on getting out of bed and onto one's feet, a large proportion of the circulating blood would pool in the vessels of the legs and abdominal organs, causing a profound fall in BP. This can happen in certain illnesses that affect the ANS (see Chapter 12, p112) and occasionally when taking certain medications for hypertension.

> When the brain is starved of blood, people experience 'greying out' or even 'blacking out'

Most people have felt the sensation of 'greying out' or even 'blacking out' when the brain is starved of blood. This can occur when the body is subjected to an enhanced gravitational force, as experienced by aerobatic pilots and fair-ground roller coaster riders. During prolonged standing, when the leg muscles are not pumping the blood back up to the heart efficiently, greying or blacking out is sometimes seen.

Although the initial pooling of blood in the lower extremities is equivalent to the loss of half a litre of blood, under normal circum-stances it is countered by a reflex initiated by the pressure-sensitive **baroceptors**. The baroceptors are located in the aorta and carotid arteries.

> Baroceptors are pressure-sensitive and detect sudden drops in blood pressure. They can be oversensitive to high or normal pressures in older people

When the baroceptors detect a slight drop in the BP, nervous impulses are relayed through the cranial nerves to the brain stem. Here the cranial nerves connect with other nerve cells that control the ANS. Sympathetic impulses are transmitted down to the heart and blood vessels and the result is to increase:

❖ the heart rate

❖ the force of the heart's contractions

❖ the peripheral resistance.

These changes happen within a minute of standing up.

There are many causes of sudden loss or clouding of consciousness. The ordinary 'faint', known as a **vasovagal attack**, is generally due to overactivity of the parasympathetic system. The parasympathetic system is usually mediated through the neurotransmitter acetylcholine and it slows the heart down. In some people, especially the elderly, the baroceptor reflex can be oversensitive to high or even normal pressures, triggering a parasympathetic surge to the heart and switching off the sympathetic drive to the arterioles.

Exercise

The body's response to exertion is to increase the sympathetic drive and the output of adrenaline. The results include:

❖ vasodilatation in the skeletal (voluntary) muscles

❖ vasoconstriction in the gut and kidney to balance the fall in the periph-eral resistance that would otherwise result

❖ a rise in both the heart rate and the force of contraction.

> During exercise, blood flow to muscles can increase by up to 40 times in top athletes due to increased vasodilata-tion in the skeletal muscles

The result is that blood flow to the muscles may be 20 times greater than at rest in non-athletes and up to 40 times greater in elite athletes. The systolic pressure rises considerably, although the diastolic pressure may fall slightly.

The external temperature

Sweating and shivering help to maintain the body temperature at a steady level:

❖ sweating cools the body as the sweat evaporates

❖ shivering increases heat production.

The principal mechanisms involved in keeping the body temperature constant depend on the arterioles:

❖ When conditions are hot the arterioles dilate to permit heat to escape through the skin. Blood flow through the skin can be increased 30-fold in very hot conditions.

❖ When it is cold, the arterioles constrict to minimize heat loss. Blood flow can be reduced to one-tenth of the normal level when it is very cold.

It might be supposed that this response to a warm environment would result in a fall in the peripheral resistance and in the BP. The fact that this does not usually happen is due to the baroceptor reflex. As soon as there is a slight drop in BP, the baroceptor reflex kicks in to boost the cardiac output and prevent any further fall. However, readers are cautioned against leaping to their feet after reclining in a sauna! Conversely, prolonged exposure to the cold seems to lead to a sustained rise in systolic pressure, at least among elderly men. This is one of the factors that may contribute to the high mortality seen in cold climates during the winter months.

> A sustained rise in the systolic blood pressure, caused by prolonged cold temperatures during the winter, can lead to a high rate of mortality among elderly men

Haemorrhage

The effect of a sudden reduction in blood volume is a reduction in the filling of the heart during diastole. This consequently leads to a decrease in stroke volume (see Chapter 1, p2) and therefore a drop in both cardiac output and BP. Once again, the baroceptors leap to the defence by initiating the elevation of the heart rate and the peripheral resistance. A patient who is haemorrhaging classically has cold extremities and a rapid yet weak pulse. Within a few hours of the haemorrhage, large amounts of fluid are transferred from the tissue spaces into the circulation. This replaces much of the plasma, although obviously not the

> After a sudden loss of blood through a haemorrhage, autoregulation works to maintain the blood supply to the brain and the baroceptors work to prevent the blood pressure from dropping too much

red blood cells. The release of antidiuretic hormone from the pituitary gland provides a second line of defence against the effects of a sudden loss of blood.

Summary points

❖ Homeostasis – the maintenance of a constant internal environment – is a vital physiological function that is seen in its most advanced form in mammals.

❖ Homeostasis is partly a function of the autonomic nervous system. The sympathetic division of the ANS constricts the arterioles of the skin, kidneys and gut through the mediation of neurotransmitters, such as noradrenaline. The sympathetic nervous system also raises cardiac output.

❖ The kidneys are also important in homeostasis. Antidiuretic hormone (ADH), secreted in response to dehydration or to haemorrhage, acts to help the kidneys conserve fluid and causes the arterioles to constrict.

❖ The renin–angiotensin system, also largely activated in the kidneys, exerts similar effects to ADH.

❖ There are important reflexes, mediated through the sympathetic nervous system and baroceptors, which protect us from catastrophic falls in blood pressure, eg when standing up quickly.

❖ The mechanism of autoregulation protects the blood supply to vital organs, notably the brain, at the expense of less immediately critical parts of the body.

❖ Some familiarity with the way the body controls the blood pressure is necessary if the actions of the drugs available for the treatment of high blood pressure are to be understood.

Chapter Three

How is the blood pressure measured?

Having one's blood pressure (BP) measured is a familiar part of a visit to the GP or hospital, and an inescapable part of routine medical examinations. The technique used to measure BP is not straightforward – attention to detail is required if reliable results are to

> Blood pressure measurement is a routine part of every medical examination and there are various monitors and machines available for taking the readings

be achieved. There are different types of measuring device available and an increasing number of people now take their own readings at home. Many surgeries also have sophisticated instruments for monitoring the BP over a 24-hour period.

What are the principles of BP measurement?

The ritual of a doctor or nurse wrapping a piece of cloth around the patient's arm, then studying a numbered scale while intently listening to 'who-knows-what' is an image that remains central to medicine today.

❖ Does measuring the blood pressure really require such concentration and apparent wizardry?

❖ Have you ever wondered what they are actually doing?

❖ What are they listening for?

Measuring the pressure in a tyre requires direct access to the air inside the tyre via a valve. Such direct pressure measurements can be made in humans, but are difficult, occasionally dangerous and, more importantly, painful! For this reason the blood pressure, which is a measurement of the pressure inside the main arteries, is measured indirectly.

Blood pressure measurement is carried out by compressing the arm until the main artery (the **brachial artery**) is squeezed shut – the artery walls are forced together and blood is squeezed out of that section of the artery. At this point the

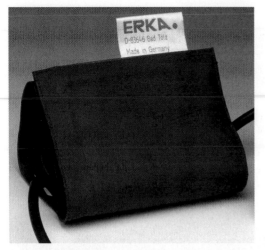

Figure 3.1 The bladder inside the cuff of a blood pressure measuring device. Image courtesy of PMS Instruments.

artery is **collapsed**. Readings are actually taken when the compression is being relaxed and the artery refills with blood.

All methods of indirect BP measurement compress the arm by means of a rubber bag (**bladder**) inside a cloth (**cuff**), which is placed around the upper arm (Figure 3.1). Tubing connects the bladder to an 'inflation–deflation device' which can vary the pressure inside the bladder and therefore around the upper arm. The bladder is also connected to a device that can measure pressure.

The systolic and diastolic blood pressures (SBP/DBP) were explained in Chapter 1:

❖ The SBP is measured by finding the lowest pressure that will maintain the artery in a collapsed state, even during systole when the heart is pumping more blood into the arterial circulation, thereby pushing up the pressure.

❖ The DBP measurement is the lowest pressure that keeps the artery squeezed shut during diastole (the time when the heart is resting and the blood is draining into the capillaries), but not during systole (when the SBP forces blood through the artery, briefly reopening it before the next diastole).

As the pressure in the cuff is lowered, the artery is able to open during systole, but then collapses again during diastole. This can be heard through a stethoscope as a tap. The pressure at the moment the tapping starts is taken to be the systolic blood pressure. As the pressure in the cuff is lowered further, the artery is able to stay open during diastole as well as systole, and the tapping disappears. The pressure at which this occurs is the diastolic pressure. A blood pressure measurement gives these two pressures, in this order, separated by a slash, for example '120/80'.

> Blood pressure measurements are noted as the systolic BP/diastolic BP and are recorded in mmHg – height that mercury gets pushed up a glass tube

Manual measurement of blood pressure

Manual BP measurement is so called as the pressure in the cuff is changed and read manually. The inflation–deflation device, which alters the pressure around the arm, is composed of a rubber bulb which is manually pumped. The device contains two valves (Figure 3.2):

❖ a one-way valve that can push air into the bladder

❖ a control-release valve that can let air out in a slow and controlled manner.

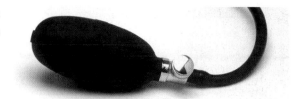

Figure 3.2 The bulb and control-release valve in a manual blood pressure device. Image courtesy of PMS Instruments.

There are two manual pressure-reading devices:

❖ the **mercury sphygmomanometer**

❖ the **aneroid sphygmomanometer**.

The mercury sphygmomano-meter (Figure 3.3) was invented in the 19th century and is therefore the original device. It came into widespread use after Nikolai Korot-koff, a Russian army surgeon, dis-covered and described the 'tapping' sounds mentioned previously. The pressure exerted on the arm by the bladder is indicated by the move-ment of mercury up a glass col-umn, which is connected to the bladder by rubber tubing. The measurement is the height that the mercury is pushed up the column by the high air pressure inside the bladder (Figure 3.4). It is therefore expressed as 'millimetres of mer-cury', or **mmHg**.

> The standard instruments used to measure blood pressure are called sphygmomanometers

This is the measurement that is currently used for all BP readings irrespective of whether a mercury or aneroid sphygmomanometer or automated machine is used.

The aneroid sphygmomano-meter measures pressure using an aneroid, which works in a similar way to a barometer. The aneroid sphygmomanometer is easy to read as the pressure gauge is a dial and

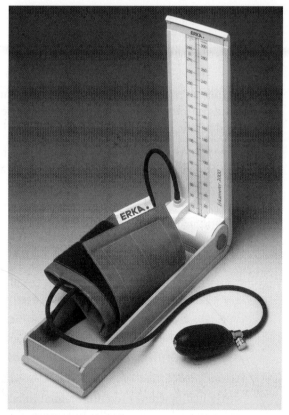

Figure 3.3 A mercury sphygmomanometer. Image courtesy of PMS Instruments.

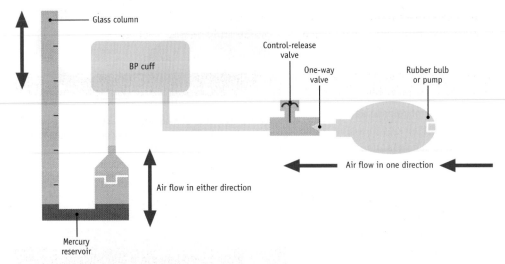

Glass column

Control-release valve

BP cuff

One-way valve

Rubber bulb or pump

Air flow in one direction

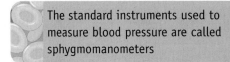

Air flow in either direction

Mercury reservoir

Figure 3.4 The mechanism of the mercury sphygmomanometer.

The standard instruments used to measure blood pressure are called sphygmomanometers

its main advantage is its portability. However, one limitation is that it can quickly become inaccurate with use and needs regular calibration.

Both these manual methods of BP measurement use the **Korotkoff** or **auscultatory** sounds. There are five sounds or 'phases'; however, it is phases one and five which indicate the systolic and diastolic blood pressures respectively.

❖ Phase 1: The first appearance of faint, repetitive, clear tapping sounds that gradually increase in intensity for at least two consecutive beats is the systolic blood pressure.

❖ Phase 2: A brief period may follow during which the sounds soften and acquire a swishing quality.

❖ In some patients sounds may disappear altogether for a short time.

❖ Phase 3: The return of sharper sounds, which become sharper and regain, or even exceed, the intensity of the phase 1 sounds. The clinical significance of phases 2 and 3 has not been established.

❖ Phase 4: Hear distinct, abrupt, muffling sounds which become soft and blowing in quality.

❖ Phase 5: The point at which all sounds finally disappear is the diastolic pressure.

Manual machines require manual inflation of the cuff. The pressure that the cuff is raised to is usually not more than 200 mmHg. It may cause slight discomfort but to cause an injury, it would need to be above 300 mmHg. The cuff is then slowly released – the auscultatory sounds are listened to with a **stethoscope**, and the pressure is observed when phases one and five are reached.

Automated machines

The mercury and aneroid sphygmomanometers have limitations:

❖ They can become inaccurate and require regular recalibration.

❖ Mercury is toxic and is likely to be banned from use.

❖ Manual BP measurement is susceptible to 'observer error'; for example, the person measuring the BP may tend to record the blood pressure to the nearest 0 or 5 mmHg. This 'digit preference' may be significant, particularly in patients with borderline BP.

❖ One-off surgery readings may have less relevance than the representation of someone's BP that can be obtained on repeated occasions.

For these reasons, the mercury sphygmomanometer may disappear from use.

Hospitals tend to use automated blood pressure monitors more frequently as they can provide rapid and reliable BP measurements (Figure 3.5). This trend is now extending

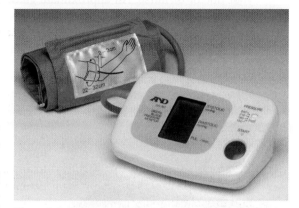

Figure 3.5 An automated blood pressure machine. Image courtesy of A&D Instruments.

to general practice. The next step that is becoming increasingly popular is for people to have similar machines at home, so that they can obtain their own BP readings.

Automated machines usually use an automated inflation–deflation device and rely on either:

❖ the detection of Korotkoff sounds by a microphone

❖ the detection of arterial blood flow by **ultrasound** or **oscillometry**.

However, the most important point about home BP monitors is that most of the devices have not been independently validated for long-term accuracy. This is particu-

> Automated blood pressure monitors can give rapid and accurate readings in the comfort of your own home – the British Hypertension Society provides a regularly updated list of automated monitors that have been thoroughly tested for efficiency and accuracy

larly important if your doctor is relying on your home readings to guide the treatment of your hypertension.

The British Hypertension Society has developed a protocol for testing automated BP monitors. It produces an up-to-date list of monitors that have published evidence that they can meet the requirements of this protocol (see: http://www.hyp.ac.uk/bhs). If you are thinking about buying a BP monitor, it is advisable to use this list until an industry standard is agreed.

> Home blood pressure readings are almost always lower than readings taken in the surgery by your GP or nurse. The target BP at home should therefore be lower

Finally, it is important to note that BP readings taken at home are almost always lower than readings taken by your doctor or nurse. An approximate guide that can be used to equate the two readings is to add 12/7 mmHg (12 to the systolic BP and 7 to the diastolic BP) to the home reading. For this reason, the 'target' home BP readings you may be aiming for should be lower than your 'target' surgery readings.

Ambulatory blood pressure monitors

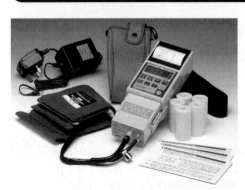

Figure 3.6 An ambulatory blood pressure monitor. Image courtesy of A&D Instruments.

This is the other main device for BP measurement. It is useful for GPs to have access to an ambulatory monitor (Figure 3.6), particularly for people who:

❖ are nervous of going to the doctor or nurse to have their BP measured (commonly called **white coat hypertension**)

❖ are experiencing symptoms on blood pressure medication suggesting that, despite high surgery readings, their blood pressure is actually low when at home

❖ are having difficulty in lowering their surgery BP reading despite using a number of different types of medication

❖ have very variable surgery readings.

> Ambulatory blood pressure monitors can take regular readings over a 24-hour period. An average of the daytime readings is normally used to assess the person's BP

The cuff is applied to the arm in the usual way, but then the pressure-measuring device is placed on a belt around your waist. Readings are normally taken every 20 minutes during the day and every hour overnight during a 24-hour period and a print-out is obtained (Figure 3.7). It is common practice to use an average of the daytime BP readings to arrive at a measure of the BP for assessment purposes. As with automated BP monitors, the target BP will be 12/7 mmHg lower than a one-off surgery reading.

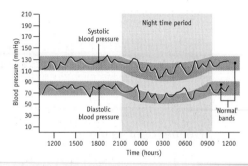

Figure 3.7 An example of ambulatory blood pressure monitor readings. The print-out covers a 24-hour period. Note: the systolic and diastolic blood pressures are shown separately.

How do I actually take a measurement?

Where and when should readings be taken?

The blood pressure can vary between readings and this variation can be due to a number of factors. Variable and apparently unrelated readings often confuse people about when is the best time to take the measurement. Almost all the evidence on the benefits of lowering blood pressure is based on readings taken in the surgery. It therefore seems sensible to stick to daytime readings even though the BP is usually lower at night. It may be appropriate to take a reading in your normal environment, such as at work, choosing a time and location that will attract the minimum of fuss. There is little to be gained from taking a BP measurement if, in the preceding 30–60 minutes, you have been exposed to:

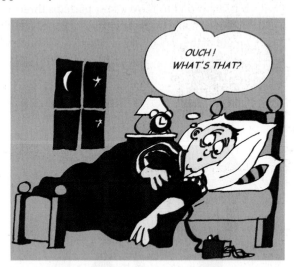

'An ambulatory blood pressure monitor can record your blood pressure when you are completely relaxed!'

❖ stress

❖ exercise

❖ caffeine

❖ smoke.

> It is best to take a reading in your normal environment at a time when you are not stressed and have not been exposed to caffeine or exercise

After a few readings, you will soon get an idea of the range that your BP normally lies in. Sticking to the same conditions will allow you to compare and observe BP changes more accurately.

Frequency of readings

Another important point to make is that there is no advantage in becoming obsessed with taking repeated readings. One study has shown that the accuracy of home BP readings is not improved when the frequency of readings is high. One reading each month is a reasonable frequency for people with hypertension that is well controlled by medication. Your doctor

> Taking your BP measurement very frequently does not improve the accuracy of the reading

may have a view on how often you should take the measurements – an average of all your readings will then be used to assess your BP.

Positioning the cuff

It is important to have a few, perhaps three, quiet minutes sitting before taking the reading. Also, you must ensure that any clothing on your arm is loose when pulled up out of the way of the cuff, as tight clothing will affect the reading. The BP reading

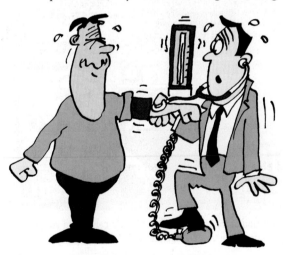

should be similar on both arms. It may be worth checking this on one occasion prior to deciding which arm you find easier to wrap the cuff over. A difference of more than 20/10 (ie either 20 mmHg systolic or 10 mmHg diastolic) between the arms, which is noted on three separate occasions, should be reported to your doctor. After this initial trial, the same arm should be used in order to observe changes in your BP more accurately. This should be the arm that shows a higher BP.

The cuff must be at about the same level as the heart, which is approximately in the centre of the

'Your blood pressure is so high I can't get above it'

chest. This can be achieved by resting the arm horizontally on a surface, such as a table (Figure 3.8).

The cuff is placed around the upper arm and is secured by Velcro, or occasionally by tucking in a tapering end. The centre of the bladder should lie over the artery; the cuff may have an indicator, such as a labelled mark, to demonstrate this. There is one important point concerning the cuff, particularly for people who are muscular or overweight. The bladder must extend around at least 80% of the circumference of the upper arm (Table 3.1) – if it is too small, the pressure will be overestimated. Most cuffs have a marked range that the end must lie inside when they are snugly (but not tightly) wrapped around the upper arm.

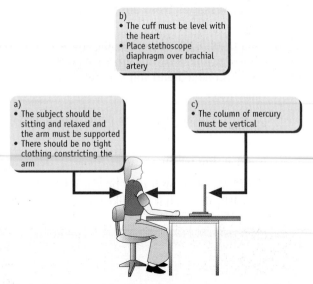

Figure 3.8 How to take a blood pressure measurement. Note: the cuff is level with the heart.

Some automated machines are placed around the wrist. These must be used with care; you must ensure that the wrist is resting on a surface level with the heart and also that you are warm, as having cold hands will affect the reading.

Assuming that you have an automated machine, it is now simply a matter of pressing the correct button. The cuff will then inflate to a preset pressure; this may be uncomfortable, but should not cause pain or damage to your arm. It will then slowly deflate and hopefully provide a reading.

> The cuff should be placed around the upper part of the arm and should be level with your heart

Table 3.1 Various cuff sizes available for adult BP measurement			
Arm circumference (cm)	**Cuff width (cm)**	**Cuff length (cm)**	**Cuff name**
Up to 33	12–13	23	Normal
Up to 42	12–13	35	Alternative adult
Up to 50	12–13	40	Obese adult

Error messages from automated machines

There are several reasons for the machine failing to take a reading, usually providing one of several error messages instead. Repeating the measurement with the arm relaxed and still is usually successful. Persistent error messages may be caused by:

❖ technical problems (a preset pressure could be too low)

❖ an irregular pulse

❖ a slow pulse.

In this situation it may be sensible to let your practice nurse or doctor check your BP, although it is unlikely to be a cause for concern.

Summary points

❖ Blood pressure can be measured manually by a mercury or aneroid sphygmomanometer; mercury sphygmomanometers are the 'gold standard'.

❖ BP can also be 'self-monitored' using automated machines, or can be measured over a period of time, usually 24 hours, by an ambulatory blood pressure monitor.

❖ The procedure used will affect the accuracy of the reading. Crucial factors include:

    – rest prior to a reading

    – use of a correctly sized cuff

    – keeping the cuff at the level of the heart.

❖ Automated machines may not always be reliable. It is therefore important to choose an automated machine that has been approved by the British Hypertensive Society; a list of these machines can be obtained from the Blood Pressure Association. Machines which use an upper arm cuff are less susceptible to errors of measurement.

Chapter Four

High blood pressure

What constitutes 'high blood pressure' is somewhat arbitrarily defined, but the currently accepted definitions are given below. This chapter explains how the severity of hypertension is assessed and mentions some of the factors which may lead to an elevated blood pressure (BP).

How is 'high blood pressure' defined?

The graph illustrating the distribution of BP levels in the population has the same bell-shaped curve as other measurable characteristics, such as height, weight and intelligence quotient. Figure 4.1 shows the distribution of diastolic BP (DBP) levels, but the curve would look just the same for systolic BP (SBP) or mean arterial BP (MABP) but with different numbers. In other words, there is a continuous range of BP levels and not distinct, separate groups of people with high or normal BPs. Therefore, an arbitrary definition has had to be adopted. That definition is an SBP over 140 mmHg, **or** a DBP over 90 mmHg, **or** taking regular medication for hypertension.

When the SBP is above 140 and the DBP is below 90, you are said to have **isolated systolic hypertension (ISH)**. This is very common in older people. Its counterpart, **isolated**

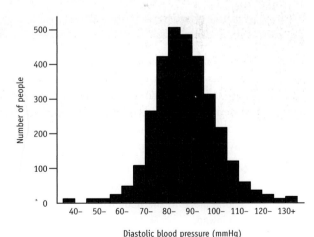

Figure 4.1 **Blood pressure levels within a population.** The distribution of diastolic blood pressure in the population follows the same bell-shaped curve as many other measurable biological characteristics

Table 4.1: Degrees of hypertension

	SBP (mmHg)		DBP (mmHg)
Ideal	<120		<80
Normal	<130		<85
'High normal'	130–139		85–89
Mild hypertension	140–159	or	90–99
Moderate hypertension	160–179	or	100–109
Severe hypertension	≥180	or	≥110
Isolated systolic hypertension	>140		<90

In the UK, high blood pressure is defined as being over 140 mmHg systolic or 90 mmHg diastolic

diastolic hypertension, is not at all common.

Criteria published by the Joint National Committee on Prevention, Detection, Evaluation and Treatment of High Blood Pressure (JNC) in America are based on the average of two or more readings taken on at least three separate occasions. The measurements are all taken under the conditions specified in Chapters 3 and 7 (see pp27 and 60). The JNC regards the normal BP as being less than 130/85 mmHg and the ideal BP as under 120/80 mmHg (see Table 4.1).

A leading epidemiologist 'fudged' the issue when he famously suggested a definition of hypertension – 'that level of BP above which . . . treatment [does] more good than harm'!

Assessing the severity of hypertension

'The higher the BP the worse the hypertension.' It is also likely that the longer the person has had undiscovered hypertension, the more serious it will be. This is because undetected complications may already be developing.

When a doctor finds that one of his or her patients has hypertension, he or she will look for signs in the body that the consequences of high blood pressure are already under way. In particular, the following tests may be carried out:

❖ Examination of the retina (at the back of the eye) with an **ophthalmoscope** to assess the existence and degree of **atherosclerosis**. This is the one place in the body where the state of the arteries can be directly viewed.

❖ An **electrocardiogram (ECG)**, which will give an indication as to whether the muscle of the left ventricle is showing signs of strain as a result of pumping the blood against increased resistance. More accurate information may be sought by means of an **echocardiogram**, which will show whether the muscular wall of the ventricle has become thicker (in the same way that muscles generally respond to exercise). This may sound like a good thing, but severe problems arise when the coronary arteries have difficulty maintaining an adequate blood supply to this increased muscle mass.

❖ A chest **x-ray** will demonstrate the size of the heart, as well as showing any evidence of fluid accumulation in the lungs.

❖ Various biochemical tests on the blood will show whether there has been functional damage to the kidneys.

These tests are carried out to establish the presence or absence of **target organ damage**. Occasionally, the retinal examination will reveal small haemorrhages or other changes which indicate that the patient has **malignant hypertension** and is in imminent danger of developing serious complications. This is more likely when the BP has risen rapidly (**accelerated hypertension**) and is one of the few contexts in which the patient is likely to experience a headache – which is a largely mythical symptom of hypertension.

> The effects of sustained hypertension include kidney damage, atherosclerosis and an increased muscle mass of the left ventricle of the heart

What causes hypertension?

The vast majority of people have no identifiable cause for their hypertension. They are said to have **essential hypertension**. Younger people are less likely to have essential hypertension, but have more years to suffer its effects. Special tests for underlying causes of hypertension are more likely to give positive results in younger people. There is a small minority (between 2–5%) in whom an underlying cause is discovered.

> People who do not appear to have a specific cause for their hypertension are said to have 'essential hypertension'

Essential hypertension

In this context, the word 'essential' means that we really do not know what causes the hypertension. It seems likely that there are several contributing factors.

Age
In the western world, hypertension is strikingly **age related**. Before hypertension can be accepted as an inescapable consequence of ageing, it has to be a characteristic

noted in all the ageing members of the species; otherwise it is simply a problem which becomes increasingly prevalent with advancing years. However, there are a number of populations that have been studied – mainly located in very rural or jungle-clad, undeveloped parts of South America, southern Africa, Australia, Polynesia and China – who do not show this rise in BP with age. As soon as these people migrate to cities, the relationship between their age and BP rapidly assumes the pattern seen in the host population.

Environmental factors

Many **environmental factors** affect westernized societies. These include:

- ❖ diet, particularly a high intake of **salt**
- ❖ lack of exercise – a sedentary lifestyle
- ❖ cigarette smoking
- ❖ alcohol (although also common in undeveloped societies)
- ❖ high saturated fat intake
- ❖ tendency to be overweight
- ❖ stress, possibly related to overcrowding and noise.

> High salt intake, being overweight, sedentary lifestyle and high alcohol consumption are the key factors associated with hypertension in western societies

Psychosocial stress

The role played by **psychosocial stress** was emphasized by a study carried out over 20 years on a secluded order of Italian nuns. When compared with their contemporaries who had remained in the outside world, the nuns' BPs were 30 mmHg lower at the end of the study; this could not be explained in terms of body weight, diet or the effects of child-bearing.

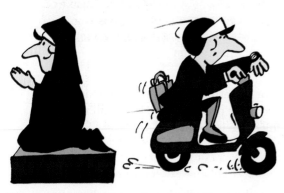

'The secluded life of a nun results in a lower blood pressure than her more worldly twin sister'

More recently, 2300 Californian adults were assessed in 1974 and again 20 years later. Job insecurity, unemployment and poor performance at work were the main predictors of hypertension in men, and low status at work was the main predictor in women. An even more recent study suggests that people who live near airports are prone to hypertension – particularly those who have normal hearing! It appears that stress leads to increased activity by the sympathetic nervous system.

Birth weight

A leading epidemiologist from Southampton, UK, has compiled data that show that **low birth-weight** babies are more likely to develop hypertension in later life, especially if the placenta was comparatively large. A person's health during middle age may therefore be a reflection of the nutritional status of their mother.

Genetic factors

It is almost certain that **genetic** and **racial** influences may contribute to the development of hypertension. However, if there is a familial tendency to hypertension in humans, a number of different genes will be involved.

There are no clear-cut racial differences in the prevalence of hypertension, although there is a suggestion that black people are more susceptible to both hypertension and its complications. Hypertension is more common in young women than in young men, although this difference disappears in later life; women may also have a slightly increased risk of the associated complications.

There is a common association of cardiovascular risk factors which has become known as 'syndrome X': as well as essential hypertension it includes:

❖ obesity

❖ a raised level of lipids (fats) in the blood

❖ 'Type II' diabetes [now often termed 'maturity-onset' or 'non-insulin-dependent diabetes mellitus' (NIDDM)]. In these people, insulin production is increased but body tissues are resistant to its effects.

It has been suggested that this combination of disorders might be due to an as yet unidentified 'thrifty' gene, which, in prehistoric times, allowed a person to lay down stores of fat in times of plenty for use in times of famine.

Another gene may influence the synthesis of angiotensinogen (see Chapter 2, p15) and thereby predispose to essential hypertension and pregnancy-induced hypertension. This could affect the BP response to a low-salt diet and certain drugs.

Mechanisms of essential hypertension

There are several possible mechanisms, including overactivity of the sympathetic nervous system leading to a raised cardiac output and raised peripheral resistance. However, it is probable that this explanation is too simple for what is a much more complex situation that involves a number of hormonal and other systems, which combine to affect the blood volume as well as the peripheral resistance.

Hypertension due to identifiable causes

Some of these causes are uncommon and specialized – they would probably only be identified after some complex investigations in a specialist clinic. Others are either more prevalent, or particularly disastrous in their effects, and therefore merit greater attention.

Pregnancy

> Blood pressure must be monitored regularly during pregnancy as high blood pressure can cause maternal, fetal or neonatal death

Toxaemia, pre-eclampsia, and **eclampsia of pregnancy** are, as the names suggest, conditions specific to pregnant women. Hypertension is not uncommon during pregnancy and may signify the onset of these serious disorders that are major causes of maternal, fetal and neonatal death (see Chapter 8, p66).

Renal disease

A wide variety of **renal diseases** can cause hypertension, eg **pyelonephritis**. Conversely, severe hypertension can harm the kidneys and it is not always easy to distinguish cause from effect. Very rarely, removal of the affected kidney can be justified, but only if the infection is confined to one kidney, the other kidney is working well and the BP is proving difficult to control – otherwise medication is preferable. **Glomerulonephritis** and **polycystic kidney disease** are other examples and cause renal failure as well as hypertension. The mechanism involved may be excessive renin production (see Chapter 2, p15). One of the mechanisms implicated when the BP rises due to narrowing of one of the renal arteries, is over-production of renin by a kidney starved of its blood supply. This is called **renal artery stenosis** and is cured by inflating a balloon inside the narrow segment of the artery (**angioplasty**), but again it is often preferable to use medication. A variety of tumours (both within and outside the kidneys) can also secrete excessive quantities of renin.

Malformation of the aorta

There may be a malformation of the aorta – usually a narrow segment in the chest. In this case it might be assumed that hypertension is due to over-secretion of renin resulting from under-perfusion of the kidneys, but this is not necessarily true. Surgical treatment is generally advised for this condition.

Excessive hormone secretion

There are several uncommon diseases where the hormones secreted by the suprarenal glands are produced in excessive quantities. This is sometimes due to the development of a benign or occasionally malignant tumour, which could be in the gland and, once located, may be surgically removed. In one such disorder,

Cushing's syndrome, the hormones are from the **corticosteroid** family, **hydro-cortisone** in particular. The most common cause of this syndrome is the prescription of prednisolone. Prednisolone is prescribed for a wide range of conditions, including:

❖ asthma

❖ blood diseases

❖ some types of arthritis.

These hormones lead to salt and water retention, thereby increasing the blood volume. In **Conn's syndrome**, the hormone is aldosterone, with fewer effects on the face, figure, bones and glucose metabolism, but even greater effects on salt and water retention. The hormones that cause an elevated BP in **phaeochromo-cytoma** are adrenaline and/or noradrenaline.

Drugs

Drug-induced hypertension is being increasingly recognized. In addition to prednisolone, the following drugs have been incriminated:

❖ alcohol: intake should be restricted to 2 units per day

❖ nasal decongestants containing adrenaline-like agents

❖ non-steroidal anti-inflammatory (anti-rheumatic) drugs (NSAIDs)

❖ the contraceptive pill

❖ antidepressants of the monoamine oxidase inhibitor (MAOI) class

❖ so-called 'recreational' drugs such as cocaine, amphetamine and tenamphetamine (ecstasy) may cause a rapid and dangerous rise in BP due to stimulation of the adrenoceptors.

Others

Snoring is sometimes an indication of breathing difficulties during sleep which are totally unknown to the subject, but may culminate in very short periods when respiration stops completely. Such people are often, but not always, obese and are liable to hypertension.

Hypertension used to be common following a severe attack of **poliomyelitis**; however, polio is now a very rare disease.

> Certain drugs taken for other conditions can significantly raise the blood pressure

The sting from the tiny irukandji jellyfish, found in the waters off the coast of Queensland, Australia, can cause a dangerous rise in BP.

Conclusion

Hypertension has been around for a long time, but it is still not fully understood. It is not the simple condition that the name 'essential hypertension' might suggest, and the small minority of cases where a cause can be identified are often still poorly understood and difficult to treat.

Summary points

❖ The arbitrary definition of hypertension that has been adopted is a systolic pressure over 140 mmHg or a diastolic pressure over 90 mmHg, under strictly defined conditions or taking regular medication for hypertension.

❖ It is important to seek evidence of target organ damage resulting from hypertension. This might be found in the heart, kidneys or retinal blood vessels.

❖ In ≥95% of cases, hypertension is of the 'essential' variety in which no cause can be identified – genetic factors probably play a part and environmental conditions, particularly salt intake, are also very important.

❖ In a small proportion of cases, a recognized cause can be found which may mean the hypertension is curable. Drugs that elevate the BP can usually be stopped and, occasionally, treatment for certain diseases will restore a normal blood pressure.

Chapter Five

Why does high blood pressure matter?

Very few people with high blood pressure (BP) experience symptoms directly from their hypertension – so why is it so important? This chapter explains why life insurance companies take such a pessimistic view of the risks posed by applicants with hypertension. We describe the extremely damaging effect that hypertension has on the arteries and the knock-on effects on several vital organs.

❖ The bad news is that the main outcome of having high BP is a greatly increased risk of disability or death through heart attack and stroke.

❖ The good news is that this risk can be dramatically reduced through effective treatment.

Why should you see a doctor?

The one reason which most commonly persuades people to seek medical advice is that they are experiencing unpleasant symptoms. There are many different symptoms which patients complain about, including:

❖ pain

❖ breathlessness

❖ itching

❖ difficulty sleeping

❖ constipation

❖ cough

❖ problems with swallowing

❖ deteriorating vision or hearing

❖ fatigue

❖ loss of appetite

❖ poor coordination.

All of these symptoms will require deeper analysis. However, mild to moderate hypertension without complications produces none of these symptoms: it is **asymptomatic**. This poses two main difficulties for doctors:

❖ patients are highly unlikely to attend the surgery saying 'I'm worried about my blood pressure, it seems to be too high'

❖ you cannot make an asymptomatic patient feel better but you can easily make them feel worse!

Sadly, there are too few doctors who are deeply interested in hypertension. There is not a great deal of job satisfaction in just giving out advice, let alone tablets, to a reluctant patient who cannot understand what all the fuss is about.

> Most cases of mild or moderate hypertension are asymptomatic, ie the patient does not have any symptoms

Some illnesses are immediately life-threatening. Other illnesses, such as hypertension, pose a longer-term threat to life expectancy. Hypertension also carries the risk of severe disability, which is likely to be seriously detrimental to the quality of life. This is why hypertension is very much the patient's problem rather than the doctor's; after all, a patient is what you are if you have hypertension:

❖ you have been labelled

❖ you have become **medicalized**

❖ you are now under long-term medical surveillance for a chronic disease.

There is another long-term illness also defined by a number (the blood sugar level), and although it is much more likely to lead to symptoms, it is analogous to hypertension in many ways. That illness is diabetes. One principle in the management of diabetes is that it should become an interest and almost a hobby to the sufferer. The patient should aim to know just as much about the disease as any doctor, and should take the lead role in controlling their diabetes in order to minimize its long-term effects and complications. This principle applies equally well to hypertension.

> Hypertension can cause severe disability, eg after a stroke, and poses a threat to life expectancy

In order to convince the reader to take high blood pressure seriously, it is necessary to take a closer look at the various consequences.

Blood pressure and life expectancy

It has been known for a very long time that people with high BP tend to die at a younger age than people with a 'normal' BP. The life insurance industry may not

Table 5.1 The change in mortality with increasing systolic blood pressure

	Mortality ratio*(%)			Mortality ratio* (%)	
Systolic blood pressure (mmHg)	Men	Women	Diastolic blood pressure (mmHg)	Men	Women
Under 108	71	83	Under 73	85	87
108–117	77	90	73–77	92	96
118–127	89	93	78–82	99	103
128–137	111	107	83–87	118	114
138–147	135	121	88–92	136	132
148–157	166	135	93–97	169	167
158–167	206	169	98–102	200	181
168–177	218	178	103–107	258	208
178–187	232	278	108–112	244	195

[Adapted from Lew EA. *Trans Assoc Life Insur Med Dir Am* 1980; **64**: 123.]
* Normal mortality ration is 100

inspire universal affection, but it knows a bad risk when it sees solid statistical data as proof. The bad news is clearly visible in Table 5.1, which is based on 4,350,000 life insurance policies. It shows that men suffer a steep rise in mortality when the systolic pressure is above 138 mmHg and diastolic pressure is above 88 mmHg. Male mortality doubles above levels of 158 mmHg and 98 mmHg respectively. Women are not quite so severely affected. What is less well known is that mortality rates decline sharply with BP levels below those regarded as

Table 5.2 Mortality at high blood pressures in different age groups

Blood pressure (mmHg)	Aged ≤ 50 years		
	Actual deaths	Expected deaths	Mortality ratio (%)
185/113 to 199/117	13	2.8	464
200/118 and over	25	3.2	781

	Aged 50–59 years		
	Actual deaths	Expected deaths	Mortality ratio (%)
185/113 to 199/117	31	18.5	168
200/118 and over	81	20.7	391

	Aged ≥ 60 years		
	Actual deaths	Expected deaths	Mortality ratio (%)
185/113 to 199/117	40	39.4	102
200/118 and over	80	55.1	145

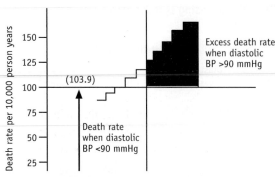

Figure 5.1 Death due to elevated diastolic blood pressure. The blue shaded area shows the excess deaths when the diastolic blood pressure is over 90 mmHg.

People with a very high blood pressure are more likely to die at a young age than people with a 'normal' blood pressure

'normal'. Table 5.2 shows that the news is even worse for younger people with the most severely elevated blood pressures.

Investigators who undertook a large-scale study in Framingham, MA, USA, followed 5070 men and women aged 55–74 years over a period of more than 30 years, starting in 1948. Death rates were double in people who had **isolated systolic hypertension** (ISH) when compared with people who had normal BP. Figure 5.1 shows a marked excess of deaths in those with elevated diastolic pressures. The take-home message is that to have either or both of the SBP and DBP above the levels indicated in Chapter 4 is bad for your life expectancy.

Why do people with hypertension die young?

Heart attack

The principal reason why people with hypertension die young is **heart attack**. Heart attacks are also known as a **coronary thrombosis** or a **myocardial infarction**. We will refer to fatal as well as non-fatal myocardial infarction under the heading **coronary heart disease** (CHD).

Hypertension affects the heart in other ways too. It takes a lot of energy to eject blood from the main pumping chamber of the heart into the arterial system against an elevated pressure. The muscle of the left ventricle will, in the fullness of time, increase in bulk and undergo **left ventricular hypertrophy** (LVH). Left ventricular hypertrophy is an increase in size of the heart muscle of the left ventricle due to cellular enlargement. This can be detected on the electrocardiogram or echocardiogram and it heralds a bad outlook.

The main reasons why people with hypertension die young are heart attacks and strokes

The combination of CHD and LVH often leads to heart failure. Symptoms include:

❖ shortness of breath

❖ ankle swelling.

These symptoms occur due to the heart failing to adequately pump blood through the body, thereby leading to a build-up of back pressure.

Left ventricular failure describes a condition that mainly affects the pulmonary circulation – it is a medical emergency characterized by an abrupt onset of breathlessness. Despite many advances in treatment, heart failure still carries a considerable mortality.

Stroke

The other main reason for the high death rate among hypertensive subjects is stroke.

The stroke which comprises the minority of cases and which predominantly affects people with a background of hypertension is **cerebral haemorrhage**. The victim literally 'bursts a blood vessel' in the brain and a torrent of blood ploughs through the delicate neuronal tissue causing massive destruction.

> Survivors of strokes are at an increased risk of having a further stroke and also death from coronary heart disease

Hypertension is also a major risk factor for the more common type of stroke called **ischaemic stroke** (ischaemia = lack of blood flow) or **cerebral infarction** (infarction = death of tissue). These are frequently caused by cerebral thrombosis, because blockage of an artery by a blood clot causes death of much of the tissue downstream of the clot.

As with myocardial infarction, the majority of strokes are not fatal, but it is all too common for the survivors to be left with a severe impairment, eg **hemiplegia** (paralysis down one side of the body). Stroke is the leading cause of serious disability in the developed world. Survivors will be at increased risk of death through:

❖ CHD

❖ a further stroke

❖ falling

❖ pneumonia.

There is a further group of stroke patients who suffer a series of minor, or sometimes even unrecognized, strokes causing the loss of a considerable quantity of brain tissue and therefore suffering cognitive impairment. This condition is called **vascular dementia** because it is caused by a disease of the blood vessels.

Stroke-associated diseases can be lumped together under the heading **cerebro-vascular disease**.

Gangrene

> If the arteries that supply blood to the lower part of the legs and the feet become too narrowed, gangrene can result. This will require amputation of the affected part of the limb

Older people have a fear of developing gangrene in a foot and having to undergo amputation of the leg. When this happens, it is usually due to narrowing or obstruction of the main artery in the thigh, which ordinarily supplies blood to the foot. This is known as **peripheral vascular disease**. Hypertension is a major risk factor, and people with severe peripheral vascular disease often die because of:

❖ arterial disease which is not just peripheral but is widespread

❖ septicaemia from the gangrene

❖ postoperative complications

❖ the consequences of a fall.

Abdominal aortic aneurysm

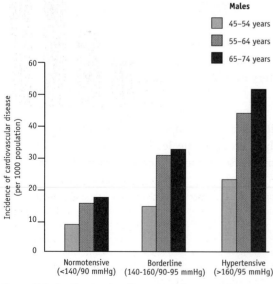

Another lethal condition that is common in people with hypertension is **abdominal aortic aneurysm**. This is when the aorta develops a balloon-like swelling. Planned surgical repair is very successful; however, if the aneurysm ruptures the outlook is highly unfavourable.

There is an umbrella term which encompasses all these unpleasant disorders, and that is **cardiovascular disease**. Figure 5.2 demonstrates vividly how much commoner cardiovascular disease is in people with raised BPs. The same process of arterial damage sometimes affects the kidneys, which undergo progressive damage and may ultimately fail.

Figure 5.2 Cardiovascular disease and hypertension.
Deaths from cardiovascular disease in normotensive, borderline and hypertensive male patients. Please note: these definitions are out of date, see Table 4.1.

Why does hypertension lead to these outcomes?

The answer is contained in one word – **atherosclerosis**. Yellow fatty plaques are deposited in the lining of the large and medium-sized arteries, so the wall of the artery becomes thickened and the lumen (the cylindrical space inside the blood vessel) becomes narrowed (Figure 5.3).

This not only reduces the blood supply to the tissues, but also increases the number of blood clots in the arteries and causes obstruction of the arteries by microscopic bleeding into the plaques. The effects are most serious in the cerebral and coronary arteries. Atherosclerosis is present in almost all adult males and females in the developed nations, but

> Atherosclerosis is most dangerous when it occurs in the arteries which take blood to the heart and brain

varies enormously in extent. The precise mechanism by which hypertension leads to atherosclerosis is undergoing intensive research.

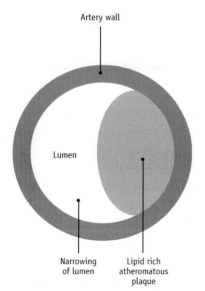

Figure 5.3 Atheroma formation. Formation of an atheromatous plaque causing the lumen of the artery to become narrowed. Thrombosis (blood clot) formation can occur which can obstruct the arteries.

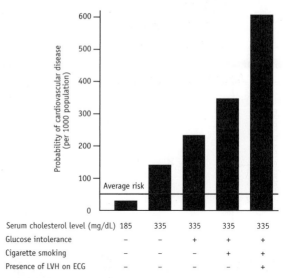

Serum cholesterol level (mg/dL)	185	335	335	335	335
Glucose intolerance	–	–	+	+	+
Cigarette smoking	–	–	–	+	+
Presence of LVH on ECG	–	–	–	–	+

Figure 5.4 The interaction of risk factors with cardiovascular disease. Risk of both fatal and non-fatal cardiovascular disease in men aged 40 with a systolic blood pressure of 165 mmHg, according to the presence or absence of four other risk factors: high cholesterol level, diabetic tendency, cigarette smoking and an electrocardiogram showing heart muscle strain. ECG, electrocardiogram; LVH, left ventricular hypertrophy.

There are several well-recognized factors which encourage the development and progress of atherosclerosis, including:

❖ increasing age

❖ male sex

❖ smoking

❖ diabetes

❖ hypertension

❖ high cholesterol level

❖ sedentary lifestyle

❖ being overweight.

Some of these factors are more easily corrected than others and several of them quite commonly co-exist – when this occurs their malignant effects are multiplied accordingly (Figure 5.4).

Coronary heart disease and cerebrovascular disease

Figure 5.5 shows graphically how the risks for both these 'events' rise with increasing blood pressure. These data, collated from over 400,000 individuals, show that the risk of stroke rises more steeply than the risk of CHD; but it should

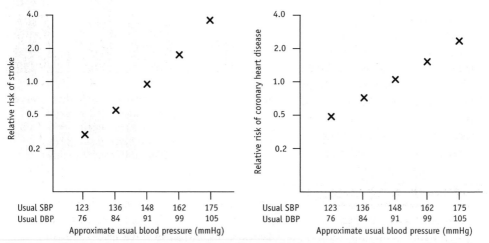

Figure 5.5 The risk of stroke and coronary heart disease with increasing blood pressure. The risk of stroke and coronary heart disease increases as the levels of both systolic and diastolic BP rise. DBP, diastolic blood pressure; SBP, systolic blood pressure.

be kept in mind that there are more cases of CHD than stroke. Although a stroke clearly is an 'event', CHD is not. What is usually meant is that CHD makes itself felt through a more-or-less sudden event, such as:

❖ a myocardial infarction

❖ sudden death which the pathologist subsequently decides was due to CHD

❖ the onset of angina

❖ left ventricular failure.

> If you are aged over 45 years it is claimed that there is a 40% rise in risk of having a stroke with each 6 mmHg increase in blood pressure

The gravity of the risk can be judged from the claim that people who have hypertension and are over the age of 45 have double the chance of suffering a stroke. There is a 40% increase in risk of stroke with every 6 mmHg rise in pressure.

Systolic and diastolic pressure – which matters more?

There is usually a strong correlation between the systolic and diastolic pressures. In the Framingham study it was found that for every 1 mmHg rise in the diastolic blood pressure (DBP), there was an average 1.86 mmHg rise in the systolic blood pressure (SBP). In other words, it remains unclear whether they are both risk factors independently of each other, or whether they seem to be risk factors because they are linked.

Traditional teaching has always stated that the DBP is more important. There is plenty of evidence that it has an important influence on mortality and cardiovascular disease. There is also no doubt that ISH is a potentially

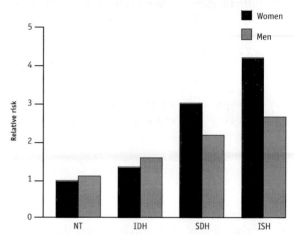

Figure 5.6 Risk of cardiovascular disease in the presence of different forms of hypertension. Relative risk of cardiovascular disease (normal = 1) of subjects with normal pressures (NT), isolated diastolic hypertension (IDH), systolic–diastolic hypertension (SDH) and isolated systolic hypertension (ISH).

lethal condition, and current opinion is that a raised SBP may predict all types of cardiovascular events (particularly stroke) better than the DBP. **Isolated diastolic hypertension** is uncommon, so there is correspondingly less evidence concerning its long-term consequences.

Figure 5.6 reinforces the earlier statement that all forms of elevated BP are seriously bad for the health.

Does treatment work?

When discussing hypertension, there is a famous 'rule of halves':

❖ about half of the people with hypertension know they have it

> Reducing your blood pressure to a safe level can significantly lower the chance of having a stroke or heart attack

> Every 10/5 mmHg reduction in the blood pressure reduces the risk of heart attack by one-sixth and stroke by one-third

> Your target blood pressure will be lower for a home reading than a reading taken at a surgery or hospital; sensible targets are 140/85 mmHg at home and 150/90 mmHg in the surgery

❖ about half of those people are receiving treatment

❖ about half of those receiving treatment actually have their BP satisfactorily controlled.

However, what is the point of terrifying people and bullying them into a morbid obsession with their BP readings, unless there is also evidence that correcting the BP significantly reduces their chances of suffering heart attacks and strokes? Fortunately, there is a growing amount of evidence that it does. In the majority of cases, treatment can be very effective in bringing the BP down to acceptable levels. But does this mean that the consequences of having a high BP can be avoided?

Several large trials have shown reductions of 40% in the number of strokes and 15–20% in CHD in people whose hypertension was being treated, compared with those not taking medication. Put another way, every reduction of 10/5 mmHg reduces the risk of stroke by one-third and heart attack by one-sixth. There is also a reduction in cardiovascular mortality, dementia and heart failure. The results certainly apply up to the age of 80 and probably thereafter as well, but the number of people monitored in the >80 age range is too small to be certain. The outcome of the trials, in terms of actual BP reduction, was modest enough: a 5–6 mmHg drop in DBP and/or a 10–12 mmHg drop in SBP. The results are still convincing and

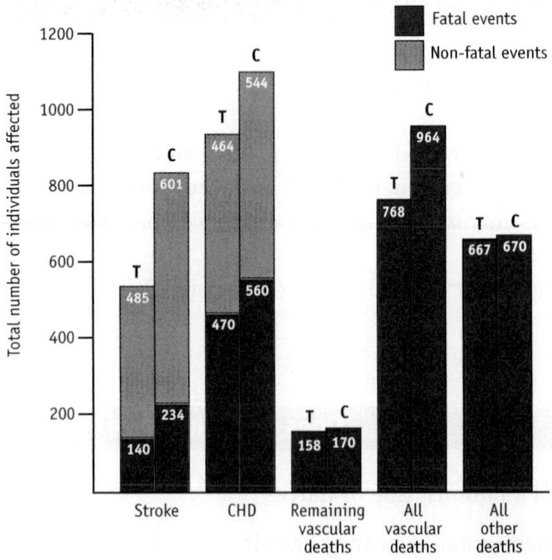

Figure 5.7 The incidence of adverse events in anti-hypertensive drug trials. A total of 47,667 individuals took part in the studies. Fewer serious events are seen among patients taking antihypertensive treatment (T) compared with patients in the control groups (C). CHD, coronary heart disease.

will hopefully persuade readers that effective treatment is highly worthwhile (see Figure 5.7).

Stroke is a catastrophe dreaded by the elderly, and because they are at greater risk than younger people, they have even more to gain from treatment. The same applies to other high-risk groups, such as diabetics.

Summary points

❖ Hypertension rarely causes any symptoms.

❖ It reduces life expectancy and can also cause severe disability; this applies to elevation of both the systolic pressure and the diastolic pressure.

❖ Heart attack is the most common cause of hypertension-related death, but high BP also leads to heart failure.

❖ The next most common cause of hypertension-related death is stroke, but stroke survivors commonly experience a much lower quality of life than heart attack survivors; hypertension also predisposes to dementia due to multiple 'mini-strokes'.

❖ Other serious consequences of hypertension include diseased arteries in the legs and aneurysm of the abdominal aorta.

❖ These catastrophic events are the result of a pathological process called atherosclerosis, which severely affects people with hypertension. Other risk factors include smoking.

❖ Treatment has been shown not only to lower the blood pressure, but also to dramatically reduce the chances of suffering a stroke or heart attack.

Chapter Six

How does hypertension interact with other risks?

Hypertension is bad for the arteries, but it is just one of a number of factors that can adversely affect the vascular system. These include advancing age and genetic make-up, factors over which we have no control, and a number of other factors that we can influence, eg smoking, diabetes and the amount of cholesterol in the bloodstream. All these factors act in combination to raise an individual's cardiovascular disease risk profile by an alarming extent.

Risk assessment

In the previous chapter we discussed the damaging effects of high blood pressure (BP). The Framingham study has led to the development of a method by which individuals can be assessed for the probability that they will suffer a heart attack (myocardial infarction) or stroke over the next 10 years of their life – this is termed the **vascular risk**.

This tool for **risk assessment** started in forms such as the 'Sheffield tables'. It has now been developed by the British Hypertension

A person's vascular risk (the risk of suffering a stroke or heart attack in the next 10 years) can be estimated using coronary risk prediction charts

Society, the British Cardiac Society, the British Diabetic Association (now known as Diabetes UK) and the British Hyperlipidaemia Association into two principal forms – the 'Coronary Risk Prediction Chart' (see Appendix Two, p120) and the computer program 'Cardiac Risk Assessor'. Risk assessment is increasingly becoming the basis for 'well-man' and 'well-woman' checks in general practice, and for assessing cholesterol and BP levels.

Arriving at an accurate risk assessment using these tools is fraught with pitfalls and should therefore be carried out by a professional. The risk assessment demonstrates how a number of different factors affect an individual's risk of developing coronary heart disease (CHD) and strokes.

The variables that are taken into consideration when assessing someone's overall risk are:

❖ age

❖ sex

❖ blood pressure

❖ cholesterol level

❖ smoking history

❖ presence of diabetes

❖ family history

❖ ethnic origin

❖ presence of left ventricular hypertrophy on an electrocardiogram (ECG).

Coronary risk prediction charts (see Appendix Two)

The charts include some of the variables mentioned above. Others, such as diastolic blood pressure, are included in the computer program risk assessment, but for the sake of simplicity are not included in the two-dimensional charts. However, the effect of increasing age and systolic blood pressure (SBP) can be clearly seen from these charts – the risk assessment moves up from the white low-risk band to the grey and then blue high-risk band. Similarly, being male will increase the risk, as discussed in the previous chapter (see p41).

These tables are not relevant to two groups of people:

❖ Anyone who has developed vascular disease is already at high risk of further vascular 'events'. Therefore anyone who has had a heart attack, stroke etc, is treated in the same way as someone in the high-risk group (the blue area on the chart) irrespective of where they actually 'plot' on the charts.

❖ The charts also exclude people outside the age range shown. People under the age of 40 years are generally at a low risk, so cholesterol measurement is of little benefit in this age group (unless there is a strong family history); and there is a lack of information for those above the age of 70 years. Furthermore, hardly any information exists on the effects of some of the treatments that are offered to high-risk individuals. Lowering the cholesterol level has only been shown to be effective in younger age groups and aggressive BP lowering can be counter-productive, causing the elderly to be at risk of dizziness and falls. The charts therefore stop at the age of 70. If you are above this age, assessment and treatment is difficult and often comes down to personal choice.

The charts are based on the initial assessment of thousands of people and observation of what subsequently became of them. Therefore a risk assessment will be based on the BP or cholesterol level before treatment was started. Any future assessments using your new lower BP will be an estimate of the new risk, and will not take into consideration the effect of all those years when the blood pressure was at its original level.

> The coronary risk prediction charts are not relevant to people outside the age ranges shown or to people who already have vascular disease

Cholesterol

The measure of **cholesterol** used is the TC:HDL or 'serum total cholesterol to HDL cholesterol ratio'. This ratio allows the risk assessment to take into consideration the two most relevant types of cholesterol that circulate in the bloodstream. These are the **HDL cholesterol** and the **LDL cholesterol**. These acronyms stand for high-/low-density lipoprotein and are the proteins that transport fats in the bloodstream. LDL cholesterol is harmful and accelerates the process of atherosclerosis, which causes

> There are two types of cholesterol; whilst one is harmful, the other is protective against vascular disease

vascular disease. HDL cholesterol is protective against atherosclerosis. A high TC:HDL ratio is present when there is a high amount of harmful LDL cholesterol and a low amount of protective HDL cholesterol. As can be seen from the charts, the higher the TC:HDL ratio, the higher the risk of vascular disease.

The TC:HDL ratio is not normally high enough to have a devastating impact on a person's susceptibility to vascular disease. However, it is particularly relevant when heart disease is rife throughout a family and affects family members at a young age: a rare condition called **familial hypercholesterolaemia**, the presence of which rules out the use of these charts.

People often request that their cholesterol is measured without really understanding how the result should be interpreted. For example, look at the chart that represents a 40-year-old, non-diabetic, non-smoking woman (Figure 6.1). If we assume that she has an SBP of 120 mmHg, you will see that having high cholesterol increases her risk of vascular disease from the white low-risk band to – well, low risk still! The likelihood that the results of cholesterol testing will change a person's risk is therefore usually assessed before taking a blood sample.

It is also clear from the charts that in individuals who have a medium risk due to other risk factors, eg high blood pressure, a high TC:HDL ratio will cause a significant increase

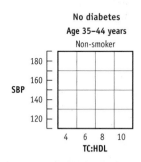

No diabetes
Age 35–44 years
Non-smoker

SBP = systolic blood pressure (mmHg)
TC:HDL = serum total cholesterol to HDL cholesterol ratio

☐ CHD risk, <15% over next 10 years
▨ CHD risk, 15–30% over next 10 years
■ CHD risk, >30% over next 10 years

Figure 6.1 From coronary risk prediction chart. Shows a 40 year old non-diabetic, non-smoking female.

> If you have a high TC:HDL cholesterol ratio and therefore a high risk of vascular disease, steps should be taken to lower the cholesterol level by modifying your diet

in the risk of vascular disease. In this situation, lowering the cholesterol level can be very important. This can be done by modifying the diet. A 10-year risk of 30% shows that an individual is at high-risk of vascular disease and so lowering the cholesterol is particularly important. A tough target of total cholesterol ≤ 5 mmol/L is generally aimed for. This usually requires drug treatment and the drugs will have to be taken for the foreseeable future, as they are only effective while being taken.

The risk prediction charts also show that people with a high risk due to a high TC:HDL ratio will benefit from having their blood pressure well controlled. Again, this is most important in the high-risk group (risk ≥ 30% over the next 10 years). A target BP for people in this group will generally be less than 150/90 mmHg. These people may find that their risk is effectively decreased with a combination of cholesterol-lowering and blood pressure-lowering medication.

Triglyceride

There is another type of fat that circulates in the bloodstream that is often measured at the same time as the cholesterol. The **triglyceride** level is very sensitive to food

> Triglyceride levels are affected by food and alcohol intake and a high level will increase the vascular risk

intake and particularly alcohol intake. This level isn't considered in the charts, but if raised will increase the risk of vascular disease above the measured risk.

Smoking

One of the main benefits of GPs using these charts is to demonstrate the difference between non-smokers and smokers in terms of their vascular risk. Find the charts that represent your age and sex (see Appendix Two, p120): you will immediately be able to see a significant difference in the risk between the smoking and non-smoking charts.

The Framingham study demonstrated that people who smoke have a higher risk of vascular disease. Other research has shown that men under 45 years of age who smoke 25 or more cigarettes a day are 15 times more likely to die from CHD than non-smokers of the same age. Smokers are also 16 times more likely to

> Male smokers under the age of 45 years, who smoke over 25 cigarettes each day, are 15 times more likely to die from coronary heart disease than non-smokers of the same age

develop **peripheral vascular disease** (see Chapter 5, p44) and, depending on how heavily they smoke, up to four times more likely to have a stroke. Importantly, the presence of other risk factors increases the contribution that smoking makes to vascular risk. For example, the chance of someone with diabetes and high blood pressure having a heart attack increases eight times if they smoke.

The good news is that after one year without smoking the excess risk falls by as much as 50%. The risk falls to the level of a non-smoker by about 5–10 years from your last cigarette.

Stopping smoking is difficult, but doctors are getting better at helping people who are sufficiently motivated to quit. If you are reading this book and you smoke, stopping is the most important change that you can make – it will have the largest positive impact on your life expectancy and quality of life.

> If you have hypertension, stopping smoking will have the single largest influence on your life expectancy and quality of life

Diabetes

Diabetes is the presence of a high glucose level in the bloodstream and comes in two forms:

❖ Type I diabetes is a failure of the body to produce **insulin**, the hormone that controls the glucose level. Characteristically, it occurs in young people with symptoms such as thirst, passing large amounts of urine and weight loss. Treatment is with insulin injections.

❖ Type II diabetes is more common and is caused by the body becoming resistant to the effects of insulin. It presents later on in life, often in combination with being overweight, and has an 'insidious' onset – it doesn't usually cause symptoms and may initially be discovered during routine blood tests, for example when someone is discovered to have high blood pressure. Treatment is by avoiding sugar in the diet; however, tablets or insulin injections are also often required.

It has been known for a long time that diabetics are at an increased risk of vascular disease. However, Diabetes UK (formerly the British Diabetic Association) sponsored a large trial, which demonstrated that in diabetics, blood pressure has an equally large impact on vascular risk as the blood glucose level. This was corroborated by another large trial, the HOPE (Heart Outcomes Prevention Evaluation) study. For this reason, good blood pressure control is very important in the presence of diabetes. The target BP for people with hypertension is usually lower if they also have diabetes – certainly less than 140/80 mmHg and often even lower.

The presence of diabetes has one other impact on the treatment of hypertension. The drugs used to lower blood pressure can some-

> Diabetics who also have hypertension usually have a lower target blood pressure than non-diabetics –less than 140/80 mmHg

times have beneficial or adverse effects on diabetes sufferers; you may find that your doctor recommends specific types of blood pressure-lowering drugs for you.

Following a diagnosis of hypertension, another frequent finding during routine blood tests is that the glucose level is above normal, but not high enough to diagnosis diabetes. This is called **impaired fasting glycaemia**. Over time, the glucose level usually rises, until diabetes can be diagnosed. However in the meantime, the risks of vascular disease in people with fasting glycaemia are comparable to people with diabetes.

Family history

There are several ways in which your family history can affect your risks:

❖ Hypertension and diabetes are more likely to occur if close relatives are affected.

❖ Familial hypercholesterolaemia is passed through families who character-istically have a history of CHD presenting before the age of 60 and a very high cholesterol level (≥ 9 mmol/L). The charts presented in this chapter are not applicable to this group.

❖ Coronary heart disease is common. Most people will have a member of their family who suffers from or died from its consequences. The Joint Societies that produced the charts only recommend increasing the risk measured by the charts by a factor of 1.5 if a **first-degree** relative (parent or sibling) was affected at a relatively young age. If the first-degree relative was a woman, your risk is only increased if she was first affected under the age of 65 years; if the relative was male, your risk is affected if he was younger than 55 when first affected. Members of your family other than first-degree relatives will have little impact on your risk.

Other factors that affect risk assessment

The charts were predominantly based on data obtained from middle class, Caucasian Americans; they may not represent you exactly. One important exam-ple of this is your genetic make up, based on your origins:

❖ People with an Asian background have a higher risk than the charts would indicate.

❖ Afro-Caribbean people have a lower risk of CHD but a higher risk of strokes.

❖ Southern Europeans have a lower incidence of CHD.

Diet and lifestyle also have an important impact on risk. Therefore people from different racial backgrounds living in the UK may share features from their genetic make-up and their western lifestyle. An exact individual risk cannot be known until studies similar to the Framingham study are undertaken on other groups of people.

Left ventricular hypertrophy (LVH) is the presence of thicken-

> Your genetic make-up, ethnic origin and current lifestyle will all affect your vascular risk

ing of the muscle wall of the left ventricle of the heart. It was mentioned in Chapter 5 (p43) as a possible consequence of untreated hypertension. It can be diagnosed from an echocardiogram and features on an ECG can suggest its presence. Left ventricular hypertrophy increases the risk of vascular disease.

Kidney disease causes changes in cholesterol levels and requires particularly strict treatment of hypertension, but some of the drugs available to treat hypertension are not suitable for patients with kidney disease. Its presence precludes the use of the charts.

Being female lowers risk, but an early menopause reduces these benefits and therefore has an impact on risk assessment.

Assessment of people at a lower risk

In the earlier section on cholesterol, we mentioned that a high risk of vascular disease (10-year risk of 30%) will move some of the 'goalposts' in the treatment of hypertension. Not only will there continue to be a fairly tough target BP to aim for, but also cholesterol-lowering tablets are often started. However, the risk assessment has some benefits for those at lower risk.

Aspirin

Aspirin has been regarded as a 'universal remedy' for some time now. It has a number of effects on the body; the relevant one here, 'thinning the blood', actually works by preventing one of the mechanisms that forms **blood clots**. If someone has already suffered a heart attack, taking aspirin can reduce their chance of having another attack by nearly one-third; there is also a 41% reduction in the risk of having a stroke. These benefits exist even if a small 75 mg dose is taken (equivalent to one quarter of a normal aspirin or a 'junior aspirin'). This effect is less marked in people who haven't previously had a heart attack.

Aspirin can cause problems such as stomach ulcers and rarely **haemorrhagic stroke** (see Chapter 5, p43). The risk of the latter is particularly important if the blood pressure is high. Therefore aspirin is not to be recommended for everyone.

> Aspirin works by blocking the action of platelets, thereby helping to prevent blood clots. However, it can also cause adverse effects and is not suitable for everyone

People with a well-controlled BP who are in the following two groups may benefit from aspirin even if they have never had a heart attack:

❖ the presence of hypertension and diabetes

❖ over 50 years of age with a 10-year risk of vascular disease ≥ 15%.

Blood pressure management

There is a range of blood pressures that is 'borderline' for advice concerning drug treatment. This range, 140–159/90–99 mmHg, is associated with a higher risk of vascular disease. However, the number of people that need to be treated in order to prevent a vascular event in one person is high, and BP treatment is not without its problems. We therefore need more help to decide in which of these people BP treatment is worthwhile.

One way of doing this is to look for signs of damage in the body which are caused by high BP (see Chapter 4, p32). For example, the presence of LVH or kidney damage would make blood pressure treatment essential. However, in the absence of such **target organ damage**, another factor that can help with the decision is the vascular risk. A 10-year risk ≥ 15% would add weight to the argument for treatment; a lower risk might suggest waiting and observing the blood pressure over time – during this time, lifestyle changes may help lower the BP.

 Evidence of target organ damage strongly suggests the need for active treatment of the blood pressure

Summary points

❖ The Joint Societies' 'Coronary Risk Prediction Chart' provides health-care professionals with a means to assess an individual's risk of vascular disease.

❖ The following factors will increase this vascular risk:
- high blood pressure
- a high total cholesterol:HDL cholesterol ratio
- smoking (increases risk by more than 15 times)
- diabetes, particularly if poorly controlled or in the presence of high blood pressure
- a first-degree relative with vascular disease that has become apparent by the age of 55 if male or 65 if female.

❖ Risk assessment can be used to guide treatment, such as the use of aspirin, and the treatment of high cholesterol levels and borderline hypertension.

Chapter Seven

When should high blood pressure be treated?

There are a surprising number of difficulties in deciding whether an individual has abnormally high blood pressure (BP) or not. In spite of the stabilizing mechanisms described in Chapter 2 (p11), our blood pressures do vary quite substantially – not just throughout life, but from day to day and even hour to hour. The effects of our daily activities on our blood pressure are discussed in this chapter. We also describe the strict conditions which should, in an ideal world, be observed when measuring blood pressure, what may prompt doctors to advise their patients to start treatment, when such treatment should be started urgently and when it can safely be delayed for a period of observation and 'lifestyle changes'.

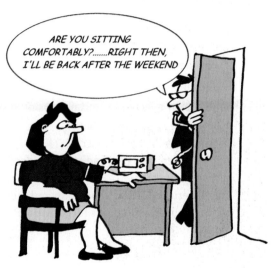

'... take further readings until stable'

How does the doctor decide when to advise treatment?

There is no definitive answer to this. As we have seen in Chapters 3 and 4, it is not even straightforward deciding whether the individual has hypertension. Many people regard BP levels over 130/80 mmHg as unhealthily high (sometimes called 'high normal'), as someone with a systolic blood pressure (SBP) of 135 has twice the risk of stroke of someone with an SBP of 110. It has been claimed that a male of normal weight whose diet is the same as humans have eaten throughout our history should have a BP of about 90/60 mmHg – similar to that of chimpanzees or gorillas. In other words, a normal BP is not a healthy BP, and the optimal BP is below 120/80 mmHg.

People with a 'high normal' BP have a strong tendency to become hypertensive within a few years and should be encouraged to adopt healthy lifestyle measures, particularly if they have any other risk factors. If we all reduced our salt intake, the incidence of heart disease and stroke would decline dramatically.

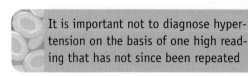

It is important not to diagnose hypertension on the basis of one high reading that has not since been repeated

It is important to identify those individuals who have high blood pressure, because if it is not discovered, they will be denied treatment that may prolong life and prevent suffering and disability. It is also important to avoid an erroneous label of hypertension on the basis of one or more spurious readings. An incorrect diagnosis of hypertension could lead to:

- ❖ grave anxiety
- ❖ the prescription of potentially harmful drugs
- ❖ the inconvenience of visits to the surgery
- ❖ difficulties with obtaining life insurance
- ❖ being rejected for certain jobs or leisure activities
- ❖ extra expense for the NHS.

Making sure the BP readings are accurate

The American Heart Association and the American Society of Hypertension have a list of recommendations for taking BP measurements (Table 7.1).

Table 7.1 Recommendations for taking blood pressure measurements

- Subject should be sitting in a quiet environment with the bare arm supported at a height such that the middle of the upper arm is level with the heart
- Correct cuff size should be used, as indicated in Chapter 3 (p29) – too large is far better than too small
- Midline of bladder in cuff should be over the brachial artery; lower edge of cuff should be 2 cm above bend of elbow
- Repeat the reading after bladder has been completely deflated for 30 seconds and take the average. If there is more than 5 mmHg between the two measurements, take further readings until stable
- Initially, record BP in both arms, and if there is a difference use the arm with the higher pressure (usually the right arm)
- The old mercury sphygmomanometer is more accurate than the newer types, but is very difficult to use on oneself

When will the blood pressure reading be distorted?

There are further obstacles in the physician's way when trying to obtain an accurate BP level. Most of the activities that the patient has undertaken earlier in the day are likely to distort the readings (Table 7.2).

Many normal everyday activities raise the BP to some degree, even talking, so a period of rest is very important prior to taking a reading

Table 7.2 How daily activities affect the blood pressure

Activity	Elevation of SBP (mmHg)	Elevation of DBP (mmHg)
Attending a meeting	20	15
Commuting to work	16	13
Dressing	12	10
Walking	12	6
Talking (phone)	17 (10)	13 (7)
Eating	9	10
Desk work	6	5
Reading	2	2

Exposure to the cold, distension of bladder or bowel, smoking and caffeine are other factors which significantly elevate the BP for a variable time afterwards. This is why it is usually suggested that the BP should be measured after a five-minute resting period. It might be assumed that readings taken without this rest would be more representative of the BP during a normal day.

A possible **white coat effect** (see Chapter 3, p26) further complicates matters. This is the rise in BP that may be provoked by the anxiety associated with a medical examination. It is also possible that an individual's pressure can vary by up to 15 mmHg systolic and 12 mmHg diastolic on separate days even when resting. Two or three

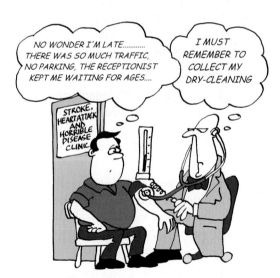

'White coat hypertension'

The white coat effect can lead to an overestimation of the blood pressure

high readings taken at two or more visits are therefore required in order to establish a diagnosis of hypertension. Only two readings are needed if the BP is clearly elevated or there is target organ damage.

When is medication required?

The dividing line between normal BP and hypertension is arbitrary, and an SBP of over 140 mmHg or a DBP over 90 mmHg is the widely accepted definition but is by no means the **universally** accepted definition.

In 1997 there was a world meeting at which 27 national hypertension societies were represented. Fourteen of them used the above definition, but the other 13 used a figure of 160/95 mmHg. It can be assumed that in those 13 countries, people with BPs between these two levels do not receive treatment. This means that a large number of people at high risk go untreated. We feel that anyone with a BP of 140/90 mmHg should receive advice concerning their increased risk of heart attack, stroke etc. This advice should also be offered to those with levels in the 'high normal' range, above 130/85, and these people should continue to remain under observation. Most hypertensive patients should initially be offered advice about non-drug or lifestyle measures that can be very effective in reducing an elevated BP, but many patients will eventually need to start taking medication.

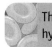

The first step in the treatment of mild hypertension is lifestyle modification

The following considerations will apply when deciding when to start prescribing drugs:

❖ The World Health Organization recommends six to 12 months observation before starting treatment in low-risk hypertensives, and six months in medium-risk cases. (We doubt whether individuals would be too impressed with this delay once the risks of hypertension have been explained.)

❖ Those whose lives are already blameless – people who do not smoke, who drink very little, who take regular exercise, who are not overweight and do not use much salt – should be offered drug treatment from the outset.

❖ Those who have unequivocal target organ damage should be offered drug treatment from the outset.

❖ Those people whose BP levels are worryingly high should be started on drugs without spending too much time trying other measures. What would constitute a worrying level? An SBP over 160 or a DBP over 100.

❖ Those with risk factors such as advanced age, diabetes, high blood LDL cholesterol levels, adverse family history or previous history of stroke or heart attack should have a low threshold for starting on drugs.

❖ People who have successfully changed their lifestyle, but have not been rewarded with a satisfactory reduction in BP, will require drug therapy.

❖ Some people genuinely find it incredibly difficult to adopt a healthy style of living. Disabilities such as arthritis, lung disease or partial paralysis can virtually rule out physical activity or even significant weight loss. Others do not have the necessary will-power and should not be rejected for medical treatment on those grounds alone.

❖ The single most important consideration is that the individual must be fully informed and completely agreeable, if not eager, to embark on regular medication. If this is not the case, **concordance** is likely to be poor, and the person may stop taking the medication at the first hint of an adverse effect.

Quite a few people are understandably very reluctant to set out on a life-long medical journey, at least without thoroughly exploring every other conventional avenue and possibly quite a few unconventional ones as well. Many people simply state that they 'don't like

> It is important to understand that although you may have to take tablets for the rest of your life, and they may have side-effects, the results of untreated hypertension are a great deal worse than taking the medication

taking medicines', and most of us would sympathise with this view. Part of the purpose of this book is to draw attention to the unpleasant truth that there are many things in life which are even worse than taking the medicine!

A slice of history

In 1711 Stephen Hales, an English Clergyman, measured the blood pressure of a horse by introducing a pipe connected to a nine-foot long glass tube into its leg. On untying the ligature around the leg, the blood rose up the tube to a height of eight feet three inches. In the latter half on the 19th century, a similar technique was used by two French surgeons to carry out measurements in the femoral and brachial arteries of human subjects undergoing amputations. In 1878 another Frenchman (EJ Marey) devised a non-invasive method of BP measurement – external pressure was applied to an artery until the flow of blood was obstructed and its pulsation disappeared. Various devices were used to compress the artery, until in 1896 Professor Scipione Riva-Rocci from Italy ushered in the modern era of sphygmomanometry by introducing the air cuff and mercury manometer.

In his superb book *The rise and fall of modern medicine* (see Appendix One, Further reading), James Le Fanu devotes a chapter to the subject of hypertension. It is entitled *The triumph of prevention – the case of strokes*. He traces the demonstration that drugs which reduce the BP reduce the risk of stroke back to a study from 1964 at the Chelmsford Hospital. This study was subsequently replicated by a large investigation of US military veterans and has since been confirmed in numerous other large-scale trials.

Le Fanu goes on to relate that President Roosevelt suffered from hypertension for 10 years – this had already caused damage to the heart and kidneys by the time of the historic Yalta conference in 1945. Eight weeks later he died of a massive stroke which, his physician claimed, had come 'out of a clear blue sky'. His high BP, resulting in heart failure and a reduced blood supply to his brain, had seriously impaired the president's judgement. The political outcome of the Yalta conference was to present the communist world (led by the also hypertensive Stalin) with massive geopolitical advantages. The consequences were to be dire for the people of Poland and much of Eastern Europe and were to be felt throughout the Far East. It is small comfort to recall that Stalin also succumbed to a stroke in 1953.

There were no effective remedies for hypertension at that time and attempts were made to treat severe hypertension by eating a revolting diet largely consisting of rice and a little fruit in order to eliminate as much salt as possible. Younger, fitter subjects were sometimes subjected to major surgery to remove the sympathetic nervous chain in the lumbar region. Neither of these techniques was very beneficial. The first effective drugs began to appear in the late 1940s and early 1950s, but these were associated with very unpleasant side-effects. The diuretics (see Chapter 10, p87) appeared upon the scene shortly afterwards and the British Nobel prize-winning chemist James Black designed the beta-blockers in the mid 1950s. This is one of the very few occasions that a drug has been deliberately formulated rather than being stumbled across by accident. Today's sufferers of hypertension have good reason to be grateful to the pharmaceutical industry, however much they may dislike taking medication.

Summary points

❖ An individual's blood pressure fluctuates in response to a variety of influences.

❖ For this reason, it can be very difficult to make a firm diagnosis of hypertension in mild cases, but once the diagnosis is established, treatment is advisable.

❖ It is usual to try non-drug 'lifestyle' forms of treatment first, eg changing diet and reducing alcohol intake.

❖ If there is target organ damage or the hypertension is severe, it is probably advisable to start drug treatment straight away.

Chapter Eight

High blood pressure in special groups

Although hypertension is often considered to be a disease of older age groups, it occasionally affects children and young adults and special investigations are normally undertaken to discover the cause. It also sometimes occurs during pregnancy and this can be very serious for both mother and baby. In elderly people, hypertension used to be regarded as a normal part of the ageing process, but it has recently become clear that older people stand to benefit from diagnosis and treatment as much as, or more than, young people. In this chapter, four specific groups of people will be discussed:

❖ children

❖ the elderly

❖ pregnant women

❖ women taking the contraceptive pill.

Children

Blood pressure (BP) is lower in children than in adults. It can be measured using the manual method (see Chapter 3, p22) from about the age of three years and the correct cuff size should be used. An adult cuff will be too big to give an accurate measurement.

Blood pressure problems are rare in children and, generally, BP measurement is only indicated in certain specific situations. A high BP – over 140/90 mmHg (perhaps less, depending on age) – will almost certainly have an underlying cause, usually kidney disease. Monitoring by a specialist is normally required.

The contraceptive pill and hormone replacement therapy

There are two types of contraceptive pill:

❖ The **combined pills** contain the female hormones oestrogen and progesterone as their active component.

❖ The **mini-pills** only contain progesterone (as do the injectable forms of
contraception).

In women, both hormones are normally present at low concentrations. However, the oestrogen in the combined pill is synthetic and is called **ethinyl-
oestradiol**. This compound can cause a rise in blood pressure, which can occur
soon after starting the combined pill, or maybe some time later. In a few instances
the rise in BP can be severe. For this reason, regular blood pressure monitoring is
essential for people who take the
pill (usually every six months).

> The BP is routinely measured in
> women taking the combined pill as it
> can cause a rise in blood pressure

If the BP does rise, alternative
forms of contraception may be considered. However, the combined
pill is an effective form of preventa-
tive medicine: it prevents pregnancy! Therefore, if the BP rise is mild, it may be
more sensible to frequently monitor it and continue taking the combined pill. The
mini-pills (and injectable forms of contraception) do not cause a rise in blood
pressure, and are therefore possible alternatives.

Hormone replacement therapy (HRT) also contains oestrogen but it is a
natural oestrogen. Women who have not had a hysterectomy also have progesterone in their HRT. Although the blood pressure can rise in certain situations, this is
much rarer, and some studies have demonstrated a lowering of blood pressure.

It used to be thought that HRT was protective against vascular disease.
However it is now increasingly accepted that this is not the case; one recent trial
looking at a specific type of HRT demonstrated an increase in the risk of strokes
and heart disease. Whether this is the case for all forms of HRT is not yet known
– in particular, it may not be relevant to people who have had a hysterectomy,
and therefore do not need the progesterone constituent of HRT.

Pregnancy

High blood pressure and pregnancy can clash in three different ways. The risks
depend very much on which of these conditions is present.

Pre-existing hypertension

This is becoming increasingly common with rising maternal age. The important
thing here is to plan ahead: if you are on medication for hypertension, go and see

your doctor before you start a family. Some drugs are known to be harmful in pregnancy, others are known to be safe.

Often, women in this group are monitored but are not given antihypertensive drugs. The risks of vascular disease before the menopause are low; furthermore, the risks to the outcome of the pregnancy (to mother and baby) are very small too. The important thing is to get your blood pressure checked after the pregnancy and after stopping breastfeeding. At this stage the benefits of drug treatment are more likely to outweigh the disadvantages.

Pregnancy-induced hypertension

Our understanding of high BP in pregnancy is still limited. In particular, there is a group of women who are discovered to have high blood pressure during routine testing in antenatal clinics, although they have normal protein levels in their urine (see below). However, it is increasingly thought that the majority of these women really fall into either the previous group (but had never had their BP tested before their pregnancy) or into the next group, in a mild form.

Pre-eclampsia (also known as toxaemia)

People in this group have two features that separate them from the previous groups. First, this condition is usually associated with increased leaking of protein into the urine by the kidneys and a rise in the blood pressure. The actual BP reading may seem low in comparison to readings that have been discussed elsewhere in this book. However, the BP normally falls early in pregnancy, therefore

> In pre-eclampsia, the kidneys leak protein in to the urine. The effects of pre-eclampsia on mother and baby can be severe

a rise of 30/15 from early pregnancy readings is significant, whatever the absolute BP measurement is. Please note that there are other causes for increased protein in the urine, most commonly a urine infection.

Second, this condition can have devastating effects on both mother and baby. Although pre-eclampsia is rare, the effects can be very severe. Therefore this condition is usually monitored very closely, and can result in the decision to deliver the baby early.

Hypertension in older people

Until recently, doctors were reluctant to take hypertension seriously in their older patients. By older, we mean people who by today's standards are not old at all, perhaps over 70 or even 65 years of age. This was not due to ageism, but to the reasonable belief that hypertension was so prevalent in this section of the population that it was 'normal'; not only in the sense that it was so common, but also in the sense that it had not been shown to be detrimental to their health. Physicians thought it seemed a shame to add to what might already be an arduous drug regime; older people might be sensitive to some of the tablets, their brains would not tolerate drops in blood pressure and with frail bones and an unsteady balance, treatment might be very dangerous.

> Older people actually gain more from drug treatment of their hypertension as they are at the highest risk of coronary heart disease and stroke

In the early 1980s, some large, well-designed studies were published that changed this way of thinking. The data showed that treatment for hypertension works perfectly well in elderly subjects; it is safe, well tolerated and it protects them from the various cardiovascular catastrophes. Elderly people actually stand to gain more from treatment than younger people because they are at greater risk from heart attack and stroke.

From the public health perspective, taking hypertension seriously in this age group pays rich dividends simply because it is so common. This certainly applies up to age 80 years. Above this age there is a lack of data, although at least one major trial in the over 80s age group is currently under way. The data we have from existing studies suggest that in the absence of other serious health problems, gentle treatment may be beneficial in people in their early 80s. Those who reach this age and are already taking antihypertensive medication are probably well advised to continue it, if only on the basis of never changing winning tactics!

❖ To prevent one stroke – 113 subjects under the age of 65 years need to be treated for five years, compared with 22 subjects over that age.

❖ To prevent one heart attack – 180 subjects under the age of 65 years need to be treated for five years, compared with 45 people over that age.

❖ In the case of uncomplicated hypertension with a low risk assessment, the figures are even more striking – 850 people aged 36–64 need to be treated to prevent one cardiovascular event compared with only 43 people over 65 years of age.

Once over the age of 60 years, it may be difficult to change one's habits with regard to diet and alcohol. Certian disabilities would render it impossible to begin an exercise regime. We would urge people in their 60s and 70s who have either hypertension or isolated systolic hypertension to be ready to embark on long-term medication to bring it under control. For people aged 65 to 79 years, a sustained SBP ≥160 mmHg, recorded at least three times over a period of two months, requires treatment (providing BP does not fall significantly on standing up). A reasonable aim should be an SBP less than 140 mmHg and a DBP of less than 80 mmHg. Optimum BP levels in elderly people taking antihypertensive medication should be similar to those of younger patients if possible.

A professor of geriatric medicine at a university hospital in North Carolina recently claimed that 'out of the 18.5 million Americans aged 65 years or older who are estimated to have hypertension, 15 million are poorly diagnosed or treated'.

Virtually all the commonly prescribed groups of drugs (see Chapter 10) are usually suitable for older people although other long-term health problems may dictate that certain drug groups are to be avoided. It is normal to start treatment with a **thiazide diuretic**, and then quickly add a **beta-blocker**, **ACE inhibitor** (provided that renal artery disease is not suspected) or one of the **dihydropyridine calcium channel blockers**. A combination is often better than raising the dose of one drug until adverse effects are experienced.

> It is usually better to use a combination of antihypertensive drugs than just one drug at a very high dose as this may cause unwanted side-effects

Summary points

❖ High blood pressure is rare in young people, particularly children.

❖ The contraceptive pill can cause an increase in blood pressure. However, this may be mild so may not necessitate stopping the pill, although discontinuing the pill will reverse it. HRT rarely causes high blood pressure.

❖ High blood pressure in pregnancy sometimes, but not always, indicates the presence of pre-eclampsia, a condition that can be serious. The presence of protein in the urine can be a marker for this condition. It should be remembered that a rise in blood pressure is more significant than the blood pressure itself, therefore the levels of blood pressure that indicate hypertension do not apply.

❖ Treating hypertension is just as worthwhile in older subjects as in younger ones, at least up to the age of 80.

Chapter Nine

Non-drug treatment

Hypertension seems to be connected with many aspects of the modern way of life. Therefore, by modifying this way of life we can greatly reduce an elevated blood pressure (BP). Increased exercise, weight reduction and reducing our salt and alcohol intake are all measures which will achieve a modest but significant drop in the BP; and quitting smoking improves the health of the lungs and cardiovascular system more than any other single measure.

All the drugs available to lower blood pressure can have adverse effects, therefore it is sensible to try to lower the BP with lifestyle modifications before starting on medication

Also, more and more people are turning to **alternative** or **complementary** remedies, regarding them as more natural than conventional drugs.

It is important to try to lower your blood pressure by making lifestyle modifications for three reasons:

❖ One-third of people will need three or more different types of medication to lower their BP, as taking fewer drugs will not lower their BP enough to reach their target level. Even for those people able to reach the target BP on one or two medications, the target BP is usually higher than the optimum BP associated with the lowest risks. Hitting the target BP can be difficult so it is important that you help by changing your lifestyle as much as possible.

❖ All the drugs available have potential **side-effects**. Often these side-effects are immediately apparent; however, sometimes people only realize that they were

Improving your lifestyle will not just lower your blood pressure, but will also enhance your general standard of health

71

experiencing a side-effect (such as tiredness) when the drug is stopped. Although lifestyle modifications are unlikely to enable you to stop taking all antihypertensive medication, even being able to lower the dose of just one of your medications can make a big difference to your feeling of well being.

❖ All these lifestyle modifications have benefits to general health over and above their direct BP-lowering effects. Many of them have a protective effect against the conditions that hypertension can lead to. Few antihypertensive drugs have this advantage.

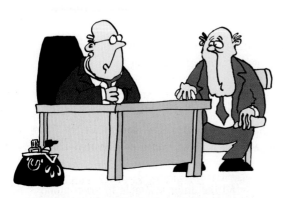

'... so, you must take lots of exercise, get plenty of fresh air, give up smoking, eat a low-fat low-salt low-sugar diet, cut down on alcohol and above all, do try to ease up a bit ...'

It is for these reasons that many doctors will advise a trial of lifestyle modifications to see whether they will achieve a satisfactory reduction in BP, before suggesting you start lifelong drug treatment. This assumes that the hypertension is reasonably mild (less than 160/100 mmHg), is without complications and that you are not leading a medically blameless life already.

Smoking

The effect of smoking on your risk of heart disease, peripheral vascular disease and stroke was discussed in Chapter 6 (p54). It is common knowledge that smoking also causes a number of other major diseases, eg lung cancer. In fact, smoking increases the risk of suffering from at least 20 fatal illnesses and 50 non-lethal illnesses, from acute necrotizing ulcerative gingivitis to ulcers – something for everyone! To put things into perspective, Action on Smoking and Health (ASH) tells us that:

> Smoking causes a number of different cancers, over 20 other fatal illnesses and increases the risk of suffering from at least 50 non-fatal illnesses

'Half of all teenagers who are currently smoking will die from diseases caused by tobacco if they continue to smoke. One-quarter will die after 70 years of age and one-quarter before, with those dying before 70 losing, on average, 23 years of life'.

Smoking is a good source of business for doctors (and undertakers!)

❖ About 284,000 patients are admitted to NHS hospitals each year due to diseases caused by smoking.

❖ These people occupy an average of 9500 hospital beds every day.

❖ Smoking-related illness accounts for 8 million consultations with GPs and over 7 million prescriptions each year.

> 25% of teenagers who continue to smoke throughout their life will die before the age of 70 and will lose approximately 23 years of life

Having said all this, hypertension remains one of the few diseases whose causation probably has no link to cigarette smoking. Smoking tends to cause a transient rise in BP, but some surveys have shown lower BP levels in smokers than non-smokers. A recent study of over 30,000 English adults showed that older male (but not female) smokers had higher systolic (but not diastolic) BPs than non-smokers. If smoking does have an effect on the BP, it is probably small and stopping smoking will not significantly reduce the BP. The reason that cigarette smoking is so important is that smoking and hypertension are potent risk factors for vascular disease, and in combination their effect is even greater.

> The combination of hypertension and cigarette smoking is extremely dangerous

There is also now no doubt that **passive smoking** has a major effect on the risk of developing vascular disease and many of the other diseases associated with smoking. Action on Smoking and Health has estimated that 12,000 cases of heart disease in non-smokers are caused by passive smoking per year in the UK.

Tobacco smoke produces over 4,000 chemicals, which separate into two forms, gases and particles:

> It has been estimated that passive smoking causes 12,000 cases of heart disease in non-smokers each year in the UK

❖ the gases include carbon monoxide, ammonia, formaldehyde and hydrogen cyanide, all fairly horrendous-sounding chemicals

❖ the particles include nicotine, tar and a number of other **carcinogens** (chemicals that cause cancer).

Nicotine is as addictive as heroin (www.rcplondon.ac.uk/pubs/books/nicotine/4-addiction.htm) and it is therefore responsible for a large proportion of the difficulties that people face when trying to stop smoking.

If you have read this far, you clearly have some interest in your well being – in which case, if you smoke, stopping is your top priority! Remember, the excess risk from smoking falls by as much as 50% after one year off tobacco, and falls to the

Nicotine is as addictive as heroin –
this is why most people find it so
hard to give up smoking

level of a non-smoker by about 5–
10 years. This one change will have
the largest impact on your life expectancy and quality of life compared to anything else in this book.

If you want to stop smoking, will power is crucial. If you have decided for
definite that you are going to quit and you are sufficiently prepared to fight for it
when the going gets tough, then you will have a reasonable chance of success
(Table 9.1).

Table 9.1: Tips for giving up smoking

- Stop completely. Do not try cutting down or smoking milder cigarettes – it doesn't work
- If your nearest and dearest also smoke, your chances of stopping will be greatly increased if
  they stop too
- 'Cash not ash': enjoy the financial saving by putting aside the money you would spend on
  cigarettes and then use it to treat yourself
- Remove all smoking-related paraphernalia, eg lighters and ashtrays, prior to the day you
  have decided to quit
- Aim to not smoke **today**: don't plan ahead as it can be intimidating. Times of stress are often associated with relapses so take one day at a time
- Cravings only last for two minutes. The next time you have a craving, time it and you will
  find that you only need to find a distraction for a couple of minutes to get through it
- Kick the habit: think about the situations when you would normally reach for a cigarette
  and avoid them (particularly following a few drinks!). People find chewing gum, using worry
  beads or holding a pen gives their hands something to do instead
- You are now an 'ex-smoker': don't class yourself as 'trying to give up' as the resulting con-
  versation won't help
- Watch your weight: it is common for weight to increase when quitting. This is partly due to
  the removal of nicotine and partly replacing the habit of smoking with eating
- It is likely you will develop a productive cough because the fine hairs (**cilia**) that line the
  bronchi in the lungs re-grow and start to shift all the debris that has accumulated in the
  lungs
- Use nicotine replacement. Reducing your body's nicotine levels in a controlled manner
  through the use of nicotine patches, gum, etc will improve your chances of success. Your
  practice nurse or local smoking-cessation clinic will be able to advise you on the best way
  to use nicotine replacement. They will also be able to discuss bupropion (Zyban) with you
- Try, try and try again!

Bupropion (**Zyban**) is an antidepressant that has been brought over to the UK
from America. It has been observed that, aside from its use as an antidepressant, it
can increase the success rate of stopping smoking. Guidelines from the National
Institute for Clinical Excellence state that Zyban is particularly useful when used
in conjunction with nicotine replacement therapy. However, some people cannot
use it and it can cause side-effects, such as:

❖ dry mouth

❖ insomnia

❖ tremor

❖ impaired concentration

❖ headache

❖ dizziness

❖ depression

❖ itching

❖ taste disturbance

❖ fits.

Alcohol

There is good evidence that in middle age and old age, a small amount of alcohol is protective against vascular disease. This is irrespective of the form in which it is consumed, ie beer and spirits have the same protective qualities as wine – the alcohol itself being the active ingredient. By 'a small amount of alcohol', we mean no more than four units a day. One unit corresponds to half a pint of beer or a pub measure of spirits or wine. Women should drink no more than three units each day because they are generally smaller, less susceptible to vascular disease and more susceptible to breast cancer and liver damage (both related to alcohol intake).

> Evidence suggests that consuming a small amount of alcohol (wine, beer or spirits) a few times each week can help protect against vascular disease

Beyond this amount and particularly when associated with 'binge drinking' (drinking a whole week's units at once), alcohol is harmful. Unlike smoking, excess alcohol consumption does raise the BP; it also causes death through:

> Excessive alcohol consumption raises the blood pressure and can also cause diseases such as liver cirrhosis, epilepsy and some forms of cancer

❖ liver cirrhosis

❖ various forms of cancer

❖ epilepsy

❖ violence

❖ haemorrhagic stroke

❖ damage to the heart muscle.

Weight, exercise and diet

These three topics have been grouped together as they are closely related.

Weight

If you are overweight, losing weight will make a big difference to your BP. For every pound you shed, your blood pressure will fall by 1 mmHg (or 2.5/1.5 mmHg per kilogram). Furthermore, it is known that being overweight is a risk factor for vascular disease; it is also associated with high cholesterol levels and a higher risk of diabetes.

> If a person is overweight, every pound they lose will correspond to a drop in blood pressure of 1 mmHg

The easiest way of judging whether or not you are overweight – and the method most commonly used by GPs – is to work out your body mass index (BMI), see Figure 9.1. This measurement is your weight (in kg) divided by the square of your height (in metres). For example, an 80 kg person who is 6 feet tall (1.83 metres) will have a BMI of:

$$\frac{80}{1.83 \times 1.83} = 23.9$$

❖ A BMI of 20–25 is acceptable.

❖ If your BMI is over 25, you are overweight.

❖ A BMI over 30 defines the medical use of the term **obese**.

Obesity is associated with many health problems ranging from hypertension, diabetes and vascular disease to various forms of cancer. The good news? 'Central adiposity' (a beer-belly!) does not raise the risk of vascular disease; however, it is associated with other risk factors that do. In fact, the distribution of fat on the body is much less important than the total weight.

> To lose weight you need to burn off more calories than you consume

How do you lose weight?
Put simply, for the body to use up its reserves, energy intake must be lower than energy expenditure; the diet needs to be examined and that rowing machine dusted off!

Exercise

Exercise plays a vital role in building a healthy lifestyle. A sedentary lifestyle is associated with a 2.5-fold increase in vascular risk. Once again, there is plenty of evidence to suggest that regular exercise is associated with improved general health, irrespective of weight. One study has shown that regular exercise leads to a mean BP reduction of 5/3 mmHg.

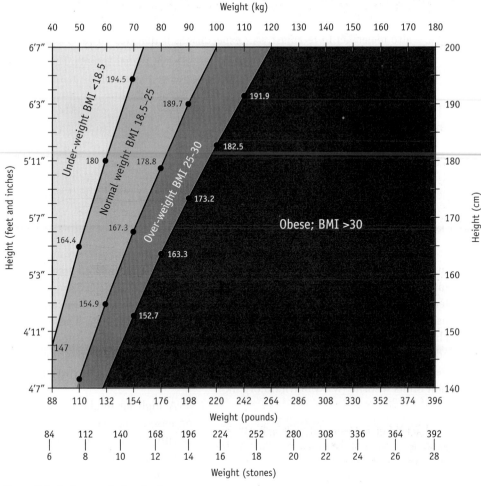

Figure 9.1 Body mass index chart.

The important point here is that exercise should be of sufficient vigour to raise the heart rate, possibly causing sweating and breathlessness. Golf and dog walking are probably very worthwhile in the elderly, but are otherwise generally not sufficient; neither is **isometric** exercise, eg bodybuilding. Climbing stairs or hills is physically more demanding and therefore more beneficial. The increase in heart rate should be maintained for 50–60 minutes per week, preferably spread over three to five sessions.

There are two other points to mention:

❖ Exercise must be 'graded'. A demanding exercise schedule in someone who is physically unfit is likely to cause muscular injury, as well as

> Exercise has many benefits on general health but it has to be vigorous enough to increase the heart rate in order to lowed the blood pressure

putting a huge amount of stress on the cardiovascular system. You may remember playing a hard, fast game of squash for one hour, but please also remember to re-adjust your expectations if that was 10 years ago!

❖ The diagnosis of hypertension should not prevent sexual activity. Furthermore, regular exercise will boost your confidence in your physical and sexual ability at a time when your self-esteem may be low.

Diet

There are three aspects of your diet that you will need to assess:

❖ total calorie intake

❖ fat intake

❖ salt intake.

If you are overweight, the exercise you should now be doing is very unlikely to make all the difference on its own: you must also cut down your total calorie intake. A lifestyle change to eating healthy food will pay dividends in the long term. This means eating food that is low in sugar and eating less, for example by using smaller plates, avoiding second helpings and not snacking. These dietary changes need to be maintained for the foreseeable future. If you need further advice as to what healthy food is, your surgery may be able to give you more detailed information. The British Nutrition Foundation also has useful information on its website (www.nutrition.org.uk).

A healthy diet is low in fat, salt and calories

A high fat intake results in an increased calorie intake and consequently an increase in weight. It also increases cholesterol levels and therefore the risk of vascular disease (see Chapter 6, p53). In particular, **saturated fat** raises the cholesterol level and so saturated fat intake should be kept to a minimum by avoiding:

❖ full-fat dairy products

❖ margarine

❖ fried food (eg chips)

❖ biscuits

❖ pastries

❖ cakes

❖ confectionery.

Cholesterol is found in animal products such as egg yolk, cheese, poultry skin, liver and red meat. Moderating the intake of these foods is also very important. Neither a high saturated fat intake or a high cholesterol level affects the BP but, like smoking, they are additional potent risk factors.

The terms **saturated** and **unsaturated** describe the structure of the molecules that make up the **triglyceride** component of fat. The two types predominate in different foods. In general:

❖ saturated fats are solid at room temperature and are from animal sources

❖ unsaturated fats are liquid at room temperature and are from vegetables.

Unsaturated fat can be **monounsaturated** or **polyunsaturated**. Polyunsaturated fat, the predominant fat in oily fish, is protective against vascular disease. It reduces blood viscosity, thereby reducing its liability to clot. You should try to eat two to three portions each week or take fish-oil supplements. Rapeseed oil is preferable to other vegetable oils for use in cooking. Soluble fibre, as found in fruit and vegetables, reduces cholesterol absorption and may therefore also be protective. Currently, the recommendation is that we should be eating five portions of fruit or vegetables each day – do you?!

You should eat five portions of fruit or vegetables each day

Certain margarines are being advertised as effective in lowering cholesterol. They contain plant sterols or plant stanol ester; this is similar to cholesterol and will reduce the absorption of cholesterol from the intestine. These margarines may be helpful, but tend to be expensive.

Salt intake

The Dietary Approaches to Stop Hypertension (DASH) study published in 2001 has clearly demonstrated that a low-salt diet reduces blood pressure.

Salt can be added to food either after serving or during cooking. The elimination of salt from cooking can lead to exceedingly bland meals. However:

❖ the quantity of salt used in cooking should be reduced

❖ foodstuffs with a particularly high salt content can be avoided

❖ the salt cellar can be removed from the dining table.

It may take a few weeks to get used to this change, but in one month you will find added salt intolerable! Fresh herbs and spices are an alternative way of flavouring food.

Unfortunately, three-quarters of our salt intake is hidden in processed food. It is therefore important to assess your daily salt intake. It should be kept in mind that salt is two-fifths sodium and three-fifths

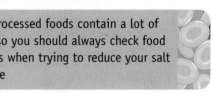

All processed foods contain a lot of salt so you should always check food labels when trying to reduce your salt intake

chlorine but food labels only carry the sodium content. A rough guide is to avoid items that contains more than 0.2 g of sodium per 100 g of food; a sodium content of less than 0.1 g per 100 g of food is preferable. You will see from Table 9.2 that

Table 9.2 Salt content of everyday foodstuffs

Food	Salt content (g/100g food)
Cornflakes	1.0
Bread	1.0
Sausages	0.5
Typical supermarket pre-prepared meal	0.5
Sea water	1.0

the everyday foods we eat contain considerably more than this. Your daily sodium intake should be less than 2 g (the UK average is 4 g).

Mineral salt substitutes, such as Lo-salt, contain mainly potassium and are therefore preferable to salt. However, because Lo-salt is 30% sodium chloride, it is not as ideal as no salt at all. In certain situations, such as in people with kidney disease or those taking certain antihypertensive drugs, too much Lo-salt could cause a high potassium level, which can be dangerous.

> Some antihypertensive drugs (beta-blockers, ACE inhibitors and angiotensin II inhibitors) are more effective if salt intake is low

The DASH study demonstrated that BP is even lower if a low-salt diet is combined with a low-fat diet, rich in fruit and vegetables. This is due to increased potassium intake. Have you had your five portions yet?!

Beta-blockers, ACE inhibitors and angiotensin II inhibitors (BP-lowering drugs) all block the rise in hormones which attempt to maintain a high BP when the salt level is low. They therefore may be more effective if salt intake is kept low.

Antioxidants and other supplements
Oxidation of cholesterol (modification by adding oxygen) was found to be an important part of atherosclerosis. Certain chemicals (called antioxidants) 'mop up' the oxygen-rich free radicals, thereby theoretically reducing atheroma formation. Examples of **antioxidants** that you may have come across are:

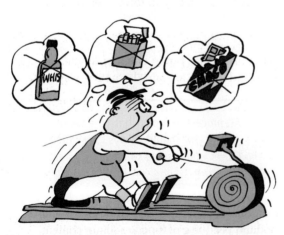

❖ vitamin C
❖ vitamin E
❖ beta-carotene
❖ selenium
❖ magnesium.

Sadly, studies of people given supplements of these chemicals have failed to show any positive outcome and beta-carotene has actually been

'You may or may not live longer, but it will certainly seem longer!'

linked to an increase in lung cancer. **Homocysteine**, an amino acid (the building blocks of protein), has also been linked to atheroma production. The blood level of homocysteine can easily and effectively be reduced by taking folic acid and vitamins B6 and B12. However, clinical trials of homocysteine-lowering agents have yet to demonstrate conclusive benefits. To ensure an adequate dietary intake of folate and vitamins B6 and B12, you should eat plenty of vegetables. The take-home message from the dieticians is the age-old injunction to 'eat your greens'!

One rare piece of good news – in contrast to the general precept 'if it tastes nice, spit it out', a recent report has suggested that dark bitter chocolate, which contains the antioxidants **flavonoids**, may help protect against hypertension.

Alternative or complementary remedies

We do not claim to be experts in the field of **complementary medicine**. However, we do recognize that many people are strong believers in it and we feel that no book about blood pressure can be complete without some reference to it, especially since conventional medicine seldom has much to offer other than long-term medication and a daunting range of possible adverse effects.

Lifestyle therapies (meditation, relaxation therapy, reflexology, Qi Gong) are generally harmless. Hypnotherapy is likewise claimed to be safe. Acupuncture has the associated danger of disease transmission unless strictly sterile techniques are used. Most herbal remedies are harmless too, but this is not guaranteed. Such methods are likely to be more effective in counteracting some of the factors that contribute to hypertension (stress, obesity, craving for alcohol or food), rather than the hypertension itself.

Complementary medicine is often poorly researched and claims of its effectiveness are often made on an almost non-existent evidence base. Trials of the orthodox drugs mentioned throughout this book usually involve hundreds or thousands of patients and painstaking statistical analysis and are very expensive. The pharmaceutical industry has access to vast financial resources and also to medical and statistical expertise. The manufacturers of herbal remedies do not

> Herbal remedies for hypertension have not been through the same rigorous tests to prove their efficacy as the drugs prescribed by your GP

and so cannot be blamed for their insufficient research base. This means that claims of efficacy have to be taken with a 'BP-raising' pinch of salt!

We would not attempt to dissuade readers from trying out these remedies (unless effective control is urgent for the reasons outlined in Chapter 7, p62). The difficulty is in knowing when the medicine has had a fair trial. People with mildly elevated

> Yoga, in combination with biofeedback training, has been shown to be effective in reducing blood pressure levels

Table 9.3 Common natural/herbal remedies for hypertension

Name of remedy	Dose	Comments
Garlic extract	300–450 mg twice daily	Widely recommended for a variety of complaints, eg chronic cardiovascular, lung and joint problems; probably beneficial
Co-enzyme Q 10 (ubiquinone)	50 mg twice daily	Described as an essential component of mitochondrial energy production
Flax seed oil	1 g thrice daily	An omega-3 oil comparable to fish oils, possibly less potent
Pyridoxine	20 mg once or twice daily	Vitamin B6 – one of the vitamin B group
Herbal teas	Thrice daily	a) Mix equal amounts of hawthorn, betony, peppermint and rosemary plus pinch cayenne powder – two teaspoons per cup of hot water b) Two parts hawthorn berries, two parts lime blossom, two parts yarrow and one part mistletoe
Ginkgo biloba	120–240 mg daily	Like many popular herbal products, dry extract recommended for a variety of disorders
Black cohosh & cramp bark		Tincture – also contains other substances

BP can afford to spend a couple of months experimenting, but probably not much longer than that. Alternative medicine tends to be reasonably inexpensive, but some practitioners can have an adverse effect on the wallet!

Some of the alternative or complementary therapies that have been recommended for the management of hypertension are listed below:

❖ **Meditation**, **relaxation**, **reflexology** and **acupuncture** are all dependent on the practitioner who either teaches or practises the technique. **Yoga** relaxation methods combined with biofeedback training have conclusively been demonstrated to be effective in achieving a significant reduction in BP in hypertensive subjects. Listening to live music has been found to lower the BP during pregnancy, presumably through inducing a state of relaxation.

❖ **Homoeopathy** is based on the observation that 'like cures like'. Substances which mimic the manifestations of the illness being treated are administrered in extremely diluted form. It is necessary to consult a homoeopath, who is often medically qualified, in order to receive advice and a prescription.

❖ **Aromatherapy** – we have read that a massage oil composed of 8 drops geranium oil, 3 drops orange oil and 1 drop cinnamon oil all dissolved in 2 ounces of any vegetable oil, is a useful remedy.

❖ 'Natural' or 'herbal' remedies – quite a number of these are recommended to help lower the BP. Among them, those listed in Table 9.3 seem to enjoy fairly consistent advocacy.

Those who wish to try one of these forms of medicine will need to consult with the relevant practitioners or refer to one of the excellent texts available rather than use this book as a source of information.

Summary points

❖ In cases of mild, uncomplicated hypertension, many doctors advise giving 'liefstyle' measures a try before starting a patient on long-term medication.

❖ The most important of these measures is to stop smoking, not because tobacco causes hypertension, but because smoking and hypertension together have a synergistic effect in the causation of arterial disease.

❖ Alcohol misuse does cause hypertension.

❖ Obesity and a high salt intake also lead to hypertension and reducing weight and salt intake will help to lower the BP.

❖ Regular exercise is helpful in BP reduction.

❖ Complementary or alternative remedies tend to be based on much less convincing evidence than conventional medicines. They are usually, but not always, relatively free from side-effects.

Chapter Ten

Drug treatment

There is a bewildering array of different drugs available for the treatment of hypertension – bewildering not just for the patients, but often for doctors as well, and new drugs are being developed all the time. Many people will need to take more than one preparation and various products exist that combine two different agents in one pill or capsule. A number of drugs are available in **modified-** or **controlled-release** formulations to enable them to be taken just once during a 24-hour period. With such an enormous range of possibilities, it should be possible to find a drug or combination of drugs which achieves good control of the blood pressure (BP) without causing significant side-effects.

> The drugs available to treat hypertension are classified depending on the way they affect the body to reduce the blood pressure

If you have done your best to follow the advice given in Chapter 9, but your BP readings have obstinately refused to come down to an acceptable level, your doctor will probably wish to discuss the option of taking medication. You should now be so convinced of the importance of reducing your BP that you are ready, if not exactly eager, to consider this course of action.

> Once you start taking medication for hypertension, it is likely that you will need the tablets for the rest of your life

Before going on to discuss the various drugs available, there are a few general points that are worth bearing in mind:

❖ Treatment is likely to be life-long. It is occasionally possible to reduce or stop taking the medication, eg if a heart attack or other illness 'cures' the hypertension. You should adapt yourself psychologically to the 'sick role' and accept that however well and active you are, you have now joined those with a long-term condition. For example, it might now be too late to take out a new life insurance policy or private health insurance, except at highly unfavourable rates; and taking up a new pastime, such as scuba diving, will probably be more complicated and require a medical certificate, for which a fee may be charged.

❖ The tablets are not a substitute for your new, virtuous lifestyle, so please do not revert to the bad old ways. Sitting around, watching TV with a six-pack of beer and some junk food is still a recipe for making the BP worse, and for damaging your health in other ways.

❖ It may take a few months to bring the BP under satisfactory control. The first treatment attempted may disagree with you – that is, it may cause **adverse effects** and you may therefore be unable to **tolerate** it. Having hit upon a drug that you can tolerate, it will probably be necessary to gradually increase the dose until either good control is attained or those adverse effects raise their ugly heads! Some adverse effects are **dose-dependent,** but others strike out of the blue. Sometimes you may have an adverse effect when you first start the treatment, but they could also appear after taking the medication for months or years. Therefore, the doctor will often suggest adding a second agent, even if he or she has not yet reached the maximum dose of the first one. Many hypertensive individuals take three different drugs each day to lower their BP. A few people will find they are very resistant to medication.

There are several groups (or classes) of drug available for the treatment of hypertension, and within each group there may be many different drugs whose effects and adverse effects differ. Most of the adverse effects will be **class effects**, ie they are seen with all drugs from a particular group. If more than one **antihypertension drug** is prescribed, they will normally be from different classes.

Drugs within a group may vary in their duration of action, so some may be taken just once daily and others three times daily, but the latter are frequently available in a controlled-release formulation. They often also vary in the dose range; some increasing in effect each time the dose is raised and others having little greater effect once the second rung on the dose ladder is reached.

In theory, it should be possible for a doctor to tailor the choice of agent to each particular patient, although in practice he or she will probably regularly prescribe two or three different drugs as the doctor will be more familiar with them than with the others. This conservative behaviour when prescribing drugs is probably beneficial to the patient. However stridently a new product may be advertised, it

> GPs are likely to prescribe one of the drugs they are familiar with and which have been shown to be safe and effective

is better to wait until someone else has the misfortune of encountering serious and previously unknown adverse effects, before you agree to take it. Within the NHS, cost may also motivate the doctor to prescribe well-tried, cheaper remedies.

Most of the drugs discussed come in pill or capsule form, sometimes in combination with another drug. A few treatments are available in liquid form, although the dosage tends to be less accurate. In the future, skin patches, nasal sprays and other means of administration may become fashionable, but this may mean a higher price tag for little real benefit. As the tables will show, it is curious how the quantity of the chemical in each dose varies among agents within the same class. This is not of the slightest importance to the consumer and is not usually reflected in the size of the tablet or capsule.

Are there good reasons for taking medication?

Many investigations have been carried out which compared the effects of antihypertensive drugs with inactive tablets (**placebos**), and also compared different antihypertensive drugs with each other. These studies have undergone rigorous statistical analysis. They conclusively show not only that the drugs are effective in reducing the BP, but also that they are effective in reducing the number of heart attacks, strokes and even

> Many classes of antihypertensive drug have been shown not only to be effective in lowering the blood pressure, but also to reduce the frequency of strokes and heart attacks

deaths. The newer the drug, the less chance it will have had to undergo prolonged, large-scale trials to confirm its usefulness in reducing the so-called **endpoints** as well as lowering the BP.

All the drugs included in the following tables are available in the UK. Drugs available in the rest of Europe or in the USA, but not in the UK, are not listed. Each agent has its proper name (or Recommended International Non-proprietary Name) listed and it will probably have at least one trade name dreamed up by the manufacturer. Drugs may have several trade names if the initial patent has expired and the original manufacturer no longer has the sole right to produce it.

Thiazide diuretics

The **thiazides** were introduced at the end of the 1950s for their **diuretic** effect. They increase the production of urine and disperse **oedema** (fluid that has accumulated in the lower legs and the lungs), particularly during heart failure. The thiazides have since been followed by the much more powerful **loop diuretics** (named after the microscopic part of the kidney where they act). Thiazides remain in use as **first-line** drugs for the treatment of hypertension – loop diuretics are quite unsuitable for this purpose.

> The thiazide diuretics are often the first line of drug treatment

Table 10.1 Diuretics in common use for hypertension

Proper name	Trade name (UK)	Tablet strength (mg)	Usual daily dose (mg)
Bendroflumethiazide (available with potassium)	Aprinox, Neo-NaClex	2.5 or 5	Usually 2.5
Chlortalidone	Hygroton	50	Usually 25
Cyclopenthiazide (available with potassium)	Navidrex	0.5	Usually 0.25
Hydrochlorothiazide	HydroSaluric	25, 50 or 100	12.5–25
Hydrochlorothiazide + amiloride	Moduretic	50 + 5	One half or one tablet
Hydrochlorothiazide + triamterene	Dyazide	25 + 50	One tablet
Indapamide	Natrilix	2.5	2.5
Polythiazide	Nephril	1	0.5–1
Xipamide	Diurexan	20	20

Table 10.2 Potential adverse effects of diuretics

Adverse effect	Comments
Dehydration and sodium loss	Unlikely to be a problem at standard doses if kidney function is normal
Potassium loss	For this reason (and for sodium loss), it is common practice to check the blood chemistry from time to time. Triamterene and amiloride are both agents that are taken with diuretics to spare potassium and can occasionally lead to the opposite effect – excess potassium in the blood
Diabetes	Diuretics may bring on diabetes (particularly in those with a predisposition to it) or make it worse in those who have the condition
Gout	Diuretics may bring on gout or can make it worse in those who already suffer from gout: to be avoided in sufferers
Incontinence or retention of urine	Particularly in those with pre-existing urinary problems – these effects are much more likely with the more powerful diuretics
Impotence, diminished libido	Reversible on stopping the drug
Rashes	Can occur with almost any drug
Blood disorders	Can occur with many drugs and can be very serious: very uncommon with these diuretics
Nervous system	Dizziness, headache, pins and needles
Digestive disturbances	Loss of appetite, mild indigestion
Harm to unborn or newborn baby	The drugs reach the fetus in pregnant women and also enter mother's milk
Low BP	Due to fluid loss – very uncommon with gentle diuretics

The thiazides that are in use for treating high BP have a very mild diuretic effect. They are given in very small doses, so the removal of salt and water from the circulation does not really have a big effect on the BP. They have a very gradual **dose–response curve** in their effect on the BP, which means that increasing the dose does little to enhance the effect. These drugs are only taken once a day. Some common diuretics used in the UK are listed in Table 10.1.

How do they work?

The answer is by serendipity: a class of drug introduced for one condition turns out to be beneficial in treating a different one, for reasons which remain unclear.

Adverse effects

Most of these are uncommon and, in general, they are safe and gentle drugs. Unfortunately, the list of adverse effects is very long and daunting if it is to be reasonably complete (Table 10.2). Some adverse effects occur due to the mode of action of these substances as they affect the chemistry of the blood; some are rare and potentially serious complications of almost any medicine; and some are the non-specific symptoms which occur in response to a wide variety of medicines. It is much harder for a doctor to be certain which drug is responsible for an adverse effect when the patient is taking a variety of different medications.

Beta-blockers

To give them their full title, these should really be termed beta-adrenergic-receptor-blocking agents, which gives an idea of how they work, but is too long for everyday use! Their precise mode of action is rather complicated, but a reduction in the output of the heart is probably a major effect. These drugs were designed with another action in mind, and like the diuretics, were originally intended for a different clinical use – the treatment of angina (by reducing the rate and the work of the heart). In any case, they are widely recommended as the second line of treatment and will usually be prescribed for the majority of patients in whom a diuretic is not sufficient by itself.

There are many beta-blockers available in the UK which are prescribed for patients with hypertension (Table 10.3). Those marked with an asterisk are available in a combined preparation with a diuretic in order to reduce the total number of tablets taken. Many of the beta-blockers are marketed in modified-release form to enable them to be taken just once during the day, for the sake of convenience.

> The beta-blockers were originally designed to treat angina, but they also effectively lower the BP by reducing the output of the heart

Table 10.3 Beta-blockers in common use for hypertension

Proper name	Trade name (UK)	Tablet/capsule strength (mg)	Usual daily dose (mg)
Acebutolol*	Sectral	100, 200, 400	400
Atenolol	Tenormin	25, 50, 100	25–50
Betaxolol	Kerlone	20	10–40
Bisoprolol*	Monocor	5, 10	5–20
Carvedilol	Eucardic	12.5, 15	12.5–25
Celiprolol	Celectol	200, 400	200–400
Labetolol	Trandate	50, 100, 200, 400	50–400 twice
Metoprolol*	Betaloc, Lopresor	50, 100, 200	50–200
Nadolol*	Corgard	40, 80	80–240
Nebivolol	Nebilet	5	2.5–5
Pindolol*	Visken	5	5–30
Propranolol*	Inderal	10, 40, 80, 160	80–160 twice
Timolol*	Betim, Blocadren	10	5–20 twice

* Available in combined preparation with a diuretic

Adverse effects

These drugs are generally very safe and well tolerated and many people have taken them perfectly happily for over 20 years. For this reason they have traditionally been deployed as the next approach after the diuretics, or even as the first

Table 10.4 Potential adverse effects of the beta-blockers

Adverse effect	Comments
Asthma made much worse	These drugs should be **avoided** in patients with asthma or with chronic chest disease, although some drugs are less dangerous than others
Slow heartbeat	Usually not of much importance unless there is a cardiac condition, but this may contribute to a degree of lethargy and limit the response of the heart to exercise
Cold extremities	Beta-blockers should not be given to people who have disease of the arteries in the legs
Sleep disturbance, nightmares	Some drugs thought to be worse than others
Caution in diabetics	Alteration of response to **hypoglycaemic attacks**, making them difficult to recognize
Pregnancy	Safe in the 3rd trimester, but not earlier; advice is required if breastfeeding
Blood disorders, indigestion, rashes	Can occur with almost any drug, but are not common with the beta-blockers

choice of drug treatment. There are certainly groups of patients for whom they are especially suitable (for instance, patients with angina or after a heart attack), and others for whom they are contraindicated.

> Beta-blockers are particularly beneficial in hypertensive individuals who also have angina or who have previously had a heart attack

A number of side-effects have been noted (Table 10.4), but their use is still recommended in the guidelines of the British Hypertension Society and by the American JNC VI (see Chapter 4).

Angiotensin-converting enzyme inhibitors

The angiotensin-converting enzyme (ACE) inhibitors are strongly recommended by JNC VI and the British Hypertension Society. They may be used instead of diuretics and beta-blockers in patients who should not be treated with these agents, in patients who have suffered from one or more of the adverse effects described above or in patients whose BP has proved resistant to diuretics and beta-blockers. They can be used as 'add-on' therapy where there has been an incomplete response to treatment. Increas-

> ACE inhibitors should never be taken during pregnancy and should be avoided whilst breastfeeding

ingly, they may be tried early and instead of beta-blockers, and they do seem to be very effective when used in conjunction with diuretics. They have a number of beneficial effects other than just BP reduction, and are particularly useful for certain groups of patients, including:

Table 10.5 ACE inhibitors in common use for hypertension

Proper name	Trade name (UK)	Tablet/capsule strength (mg)	Usual daily dose (mg)
Captopril*	Capoten	12.5, 25, 50	6.25–25 twice
Cilazapril	Vascace	0.25, 0.5, 1	1–5
Enalapril*	Innovace	2.5, 5, 10, 20	5–20
Fosinopril	Staril	10, 20	10–30
Imidapril	Tanatril	5, 10	2.5–10
Lisinopril*	Zestril, Carace	2.5, 5, 10, 20	2.5–20
Moexipril	Perdix	7.5, 15	7.5–30
Perindopril	Coversyl	2, 4	2–6
Quinapril*	Accupro	5, 10, 20, 40	10–40
Ramipril	Tritace	1.25, 2.5, 5	1.25–5
Trandolapril	Gopten	0.5, 1, 2	0.5–2

* Also available in combined preparation with a diuretic (hydrochlorothiazide)

❖ patients with heart failure

❖ patients with enlargement of the left ventricle (Chapter 5, p42)

❖ patients who have suffered a heart attack

❖ patients with certain diseases affecting the kidneys, such as diabetes.

Although the range of adverse effects looks pretty formidable and some of the adverse effects are serious, the large majority who can tolerate **ACE inhibitors** find them very agreeable drugs to take. They should never be taken by pregnant women and it is advisable to avoid them if breastfeeding. For individual ACE inhibitors, see Table 10.5.

How do ACE inhibitors work?

The enzyme renin (made in the kidneys) is initially converted into the inactive angiotensin I, and is then changed into angiotensin II by angiotensin-converting enzyme. This substance elevates the arterial pressure by causing the resistance vessels to contract. A chemical which blocks the effect of angiotensin-converting enzyme will therefore prevent the production of angiotensin II, the resistance vessels will expand and the BP will fall.

Table 10.6 Potential adverse effects of the ACE inhibitors

Adverse effect	Comments
Excessive fall in BP	This is much more common when they are given for other purposes, such as heart failure. This can still occur in older people and those with heart-valve disease, who may experience symptoms at BP levels that younger people without hypertension would easily tolerate
Kidney failure	This is principally a danger in those who already have certain types of kidney disease, but because of this possibility and the one mentioned above, patients already taking diuretics are sometimes advised to stop them or reduce the dose at the start of ACE inhibitor treatment
Troublesome dry cough	Can be very irritating and may necessitate stopping the drug
Various allergic reactions, including rashes	Uncommon but potentially serious
Blood disorders	Uncommon but potentially serious
Taste disturbance	May respond to decreasing the dose
Potassium accumulation	Can occur if the kidneys are diseased or patient is taking a potassium-sparing drug
Neurological symptoms	Headache, dizziness, cramps, fatigue, sleep and mood disturbance
Digestive problems	Nausea, abdominal pain, diarrhoea, jaundice and mouth ulcers

Adverse effects

Just like the other drugs we have discussed, ACE inhibitors seem to have a number of other actions additional to the one for which they were designed. Most of these other actions have beneficial effects on the BP. A wide range of adverse effects has also been documented (Table 10.6).

Angiotensin II receptor antagonists

The cough which troubles 10–20% of those taking ACE inhibitors is thought to be caused by the accumulation of a substance called **bradykinin**, whose breakdown in the body is prevented by these drugs. The angiotensin receptor antagonists (Table 10.7) have recently been developed to prevent angiotensin from acting on the muscle of the arterioles and small arteries. They therefore lower the BP while allowing bradykinin to be destroyed so that it does not cause a cough. These agents seem to be free from

> 10–20% of people taking ACE inhibitors develop a dry cough (which although not dangerous, can be very irritating) due to the accumulation of bradykinin

many of the other adverse effects associated with ACE inhibitors, yet also appear to be effective antihypertensive drugs. They are an important new addition to the antihypertensive therapies and seem to be particularly suitable for people who need to preserve speed of reaction, such as pilots and sportsmen.

Adverse effects

These products are still too new for a very clear picture of their adverse effects to have emerged, but it appears that allergic reactions are much less common with

Table 10.7 Angiotensin II receptor antagonists used for hypertension

Proper name	Trade name (UK)	Tablet/capsule strength (mg)	Usual daily dose (mg)
Candesartan	Amias	4, 8, 16	2–16
Eprosartan	Teveten	300, 400, 600	300–800
Irbesartan	Aprovel	75, 150, 300	75–300
Losartan*	Cozaar	25, 50	25–75
Telmisartan	Micardis	40, 80	40–80
Valsartan	Diovan	40, 80	40–160

* Also available in combined preparation with a diuretic (hydrochlorothiazide)

these drugs than with the ACE inhibitors. Blood disorders, particularly suppression of the white cells, is known to occur in about one in 50 people taking valsartan, and liver damage has been reported with all of these agents.

Beneficial effects

Recent research suggests that the ACE inhibitors, and perhaps the sartans, may have a protective effect against stroke, independent of their BP-lowering action. They also seem to preserve skeletal muscle and strength in older people and have a beneficial effect on heart muscle.

Calcium channel blockers

Calcium channel blockers are also known as **calcium antagonists**. Calcium ions act as an important messenger in the muscle cells of the arterioles, small arteries and heart. These drugs are designed to block the slow current of calcium into these cells and therefore inhibit the action of these muscle cells, ie the vessels are prevented from constricting. Some of these drugs have a much greater effect on the heart muscle than others and cause the heartbeat to be less powerful and the heart rate to slow down.

The sub-group known as the **dihydropyridines** have very little effect on the heart and have been widely recommended especially for older people with

Table 10.8 Calcium channel blockers in common use for hypertension

Proper name	Trade name (UK)	Strength of tablet/capsule (mg)	Usual daily dose (mg)
Dihydropyridines			
Amlodipine	Istin	5, 10	5–10
Felodipine	Plendil	2.5, 5, 10	2.5–10
Isradipine	Prescal	2.5	2.5–5 twice
Lacidipine	Motens	2, 4	2–6
Lercanidipine	Zanidip	10	10–20
Nicardipine*	Cardene	20, 30, 45	20–30 three times
Nifedipine*	Adalat	5, 10, 20, 30, 40, 60	10–40 twice
Nisoldipine	Syscor	10, 20, 30	10–40
Rate-limiting calcium antagonists			
Diltiazem*	Tildiem	60, 90, 120, 180, 200, 240, 300, 360	60–120 three times
Verapamil*	Cordilox	40, 80, 120 ,160	120 twice – 160 three times

* Controlled-release preparations are generally prescribed, particularly for the higher doses, to enable the drug to be taken just once a day and to reduce the number of tablets or capsules that have to be swallowed.

elevation of the systolic pressure rather than the diastolic pressure. The dihydropyridines are quite frequently given together with beta-blockers. The **rate-limiting** calcium channel blockers, particularly verapamil, must not be taken in conjunction with a beta-blocker, although they can be used together with an ACE inhibitor.

> Calcium antagonists vary in their actions – some prevent the muscles in blood vessel walls from constricting and others can also cause the heart rate to drop and the heartbeat to weaken

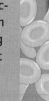

In general these drugs (Table 10.8) are safe and effective and very many patients have been extremely well controlled on them for long periods of time. Doubt has recently been cast as to whether they are as effective as other available groups of drugs in the prevention of 'end-points', which is the fundamental purpose of therapy. This particularly applies to short-acting preparations, such as nifedipine 5 mg or 10 mg.

> Rate-limiting calcium channel blockers must never be taken in combination with a beta-blocker

Adverse effects

Headache, flushing and ankle swelling can occur when taking a dihydropyridine and constipation can be a significant problem with verapamil. Dizziness and indigestion occasionally occur with all the agents in this class and skin rashes are not uncommon.

Drug interactions

All antihypertensive drugs can be regarded as interacting with one another in that they will have an additive BP-lowering effect; after all, this is why many people take two or three different drugs. Some combinations of drugs are safer than others; in particular, it is important to be cautious when starting an ACE inhibitor on top of a diuretic. Table 10.9 gives some of the other common drug interactions.

Other classes of drugs for hypertension

Most people with mild to moderate hypertension can be controlled with one or more of the drugs we have discussed. There are a few people whose BP cannot be controlled by these drugs or who develop side-effects to one drug after another. There are still several antihypertensive drugs in reserve (Table 10.10). Although they are seldom used as first- or second-line agents, because they are rather more likely to give rise to AEs, they are certainly well worth a try in these individuals and many people do find them effective and perfectly acceptable.

Table 10.9 Potential interactions with antihypertensive drugs

Class of antihypertensive drug	Possible interactions	Description of interaction
Diuretics	Drugs taken for arthritis	Many drugs taken for arthritis can cause damage to the kidneys; this risk is increased by diuretics
	Chlorpropamide	Occasionally get a low serum sodium level which can have severe consequences
	Carbamazepine	Occasionally get a low serum sodium level which can have severe consequences
	Lithium	The level of lithium in the blood may be too high
Beta-blockers	Drugs taken for arthritis	The arthritis drugs may antagonize the effect of the beta-blocker
	Anaesthetics, hypnotics, anxiolytics	May enhance the BP-lowering effect of beta-blockers
	Antidiabetic drugs	The effect of antidiabetic drugs may be enhanced
	Cardiac drugs	Digoxin and other drugs for abnormal heart rhythms can present problems if used with beta-blockers
ACE inhibitors, angiotensin II receptor blockers	Analgesics, anaesthetics, hypnotics, anxiolytics	These can reduce the effect of the ACE inhibitor
	Digoxin	Level of digoxin elevated and possibly toxic – this is a particular problem with telmisartan
	Lithium	Raised blood level due to reduced excretion
	Drugs taken for arthritis	Kidney damage, sometimes severe
Calcium blockers	Grapefruit juice	Can cause raised blood levels of many of the calcium antagonists
	Anaesthetics	Increased BP-lowering effect
	Cardiac drugs	Drugs for abnormal heart rhythms present problems with verapamil and, to a lesser extent, diltiazem
	Anticonvulsants	The prescribing doctor should check for possible interactions
	Antimalarials	The prescribing doctor should check for possible interactions
	Lithium	Lithium toxicity possible with verapamil and diltiazem

Table 10.10 Other drugs used in hypertension

Proper name	Trade name (UK)	Usual dose (mg)	Comments
Alpha receptor antagonists			
Doxazosin	Cardura	1–4 or more	
Indoramin	Baratol	25–50	Taken twice daily
Prazosin	Hypovase	0.5–1	Taken thrice daily
Terazosin	Hytrin	1–10	
Centrally acting agents			
Clonidine	Catapres	0.25–0.75	Additional AEs include rashes and nausea
Methyldopa	Aldomet	500–2000	May cause anaemia, liver damage, Parkinsonism, rashes; however it is useful during pregnancy
Moxonidine	Physiotens	0.2–0.6	AEs include nausea and sedation
Vasodilators			
Hydralazine	Apresoline	2.5–100	AEs are numerous and include blood disorders and nausea; however it is useful during pregnancy
Minoxidil	Loniten	2.5–50	AEs include rashes and indigestion

Alpha receptor antagonists

Alpha receptor antagonists block the 'alpha' actions of noradrenaline which constrict the blood vessels in the skin, gut and kidney (see Chapter 2, p14). Some of these drugs lower the BP rather abruptly (see Chapter 12, p111) unless introduced gradually, and might cause dizziness and faintness. Otherwise, alpha receptor antagonists are free of serious adverse effects, are useful in resistant cases and are often used together with one or more of the agents already listed in this chapter. One of their other pharmacological benefits is to improve the symptoms of men who have an enlarged prostate. Most of the drugs in this section can cause ankle swelling, headache and a rapid heartbeat.

Centrally acting antihypertensive agents

The **centrally acting antihypertensive agents** reduce the 'sympathetic drive' within the central nervous system that activates the sympathetic nervous system. The older drugs in this class tend to make the user sleepy and give rise

The centrally acting agent methyldopa and the vasodilator hydralazine are two of the few drugs which are safe to take during pregnancy

to a dry mouth and swollen ankles, but methyldopa does seem safe to take, particularly during pregnancy (Chapter 8).

Vasodilators

Vasodilators may act by directly relaxing the muscle in the resistance vessels, although their mode of action could be more complex – it is still not fully understood. Minoxidil is particularly effective, but tends to cause considerable ankle swelling and so should be taken along with an effective diuretic. It also causes a rapid heartbeat so a beta-blocker will probably be needed as well. The main drawback of minoxidil to its potential female users is its tendency to encourage the growth of body hair. The other main agent in this class, hydralazine, is useful in emergencies, particularly during pregnancy.

Special situations

There is an uncommon and very severe form of hypertension often called **accelerated hypertension** or **malignant hypertension** (strictly speaking, these are not exactly the same disorder). People with this condition should be admitted to hospital where specialist treatment and investigation can be undertaken.

Some people's BP remains stubbornly reluctant to respond to any drug, even when pushed to the maximum dose recommended or tolerated. When doctors are baffled, they often react by blaming their patients! Doctors tend to assume that when someone's BP is not lowered by medicines, it is because the patient is not actually taking the tablets or is taking them irregularly. Failure to take prescribed drugs as instructed may be due to:

❖ forgetfulness
❖ the patient believing that the drugs are 'disagreeing' with them
❖ the doctor failing to convince the patient of the importance of the medication.

There are many communication difficulties that can beset the doctor–patient relationship. One of the most common is the logical assumption by patients that if they are better, they can stop taking the tablets. However, the equally logical viewpoint of the doctor is that patients are only better because they are taking the tablets and should therefore continue to take them. In the case of hypertension, the latter viewpoint is almost always correct.

It is true that some people are non-concordant with their medication. Which of us can put our hand on our heart and swear that we

> It is important for patients to understand that their BP is lower because they are taking tablets and should therefore continue to take them; NOT that because their BP is lower, they can stop taking the medication

have never forgotten one dose of whatever we happen to be taking at the time? However, recent surveys have suggested that non-concordance is really an excuse and is far less common than physicians assumed. Before accusing their patients of being uncooperative, doctors must consider other possible reasons for the BP remaining elevated. The main reasons are:

❖ the BP measuring instrument currently being used is giving false readings

❖ continued use of medicines which tend to elevate the BP, such as anti-inflammatory agents for arthritis, oral contraceptives or nasal decongest-ants

❖ continued adverse lifestyle factors, eg obesity, alcohol misuse, snoring

❖ an identifiable cause for the hypertension, particularly kidney disease

❖ the white coat effect – readings taken at home, or those recorded by an ambulatory monitoring device (Chapter 3, p26) may be more reliable and may suggest that the hypertension is **labile** (very variable). There is evidence to suggest that labile hypertension is a serious risk factor for vascular problems.

Finally, what about patients who have already suffered a stroke? It is generally agreed that it is not safe to lower the BP quickly in the im-mediate aftermath of a stroke, but

> The very severe form of hypertension known as 'accelerated' or 'malignant' hypertension requires hospitalization and specialist treatment

such people are at high risk of a further stroke and it is probably wise to correct unacceptably high BP levels once the medical condition has stabilized.

Looking to the future

With so many potential therapies at our disposal, one might wonder if there is any point in conducting research to identify yet more antihypertensive drugs. Consid-erable research is being undertaken in laboratories all over the world to find new classes of drug with different pharmacological actions. Hopefully, any new drugs will be of benefit to those who cannot tolerate any of the existing products or whose BP is resistant to them.

Genetics features in every field of medical research these days and hyperten-sion is no exception. Hypertension is not a disorder caused by one single-gene defect. There appear to be different types of hypertension characterized by patients' responses to the different classes of drug. These types seem to have different genetic backgrounds associated with them and there has already been considerable success in identifying some of the genetic variations involved. It is certain that we will hear more as this genetic story unfolds.

Summary points

❖ Drug treatment for hypertension is likely to be necessary for the rest of one's life.

❖ It is unlikely to make the recipient feel better, but it can easily make them feel worse.

❖ There is a wide range of different classes of drug available; each class has different actions, different adverse effects and contains a number of individual drugs.

❖ The majority of patients will require more than one drug to achieve satisfactory control, so it is increasingly common to use low-dose combination therapy.

❖ It is better to take relatively small doses of two or three different preparations than to increase the dose of one single drug until adverse effects are experienced.

❖ Certain types of agent are especially suitable or unsuitable for particular individuals.

❖ New formulations of existing drugs, new combinations of drugs, new members of existing classes of drug and probably new classes of drug, can certainly be expected to appear on the market shortly after the publication of this book – research and development is rapid.

❖ No mention has been made of some specific drugs that are used in very resistant cases and hypertensive emergencies.

Chapter Eleven

Taking control of your blood pressure

The hospital outpatient department and even the familiar GP surgery are often stressful settings. Blood pressure (BP) readings taken in these environments are unlikely to be truly representative of the levels that exist during our ordinary daily lives. For this reason, and because of the relative infrequency of attendance, it is difficult for the doctor or nurse to obtain an accurate picture of their patient's BP. The purpose of this book up to now has been to supply you with detailed information about blood pressure and the problems that a high blood pressure can cause. In this chapter we hope to emphasize why it is extremely helpful if you take some responsibility for your blood pressure and are involved with its monitoring, and indicate how this can be done.

> Your GP or practice nurse is a readily accessible source of advice on how to manage your hypertension

Traditional hypertension management

Management of hypertension has traditionally taken a fairly standard form and usually entails intermittent appointments with the nurse or doctor. A BP reading is taken and the continuing management of your hypertension is then agreed. However, there are failings in this system.

You will remember that it is important to come early to your appointment, so that you have at least five minutes of rest and relaxation prior to your reading being taken. Rushing to your appointment or arriving by bicycle with insufficient rest will make this reading inaccurate. You may be feeling anxious about what the reading will show and what the doctor or nurse will have to say about it:

❖ Did your smoking cessation/weight reduction regime go badly wrong since you were last here?

❖ Will the doctor or nurse find that your BP is still poorly controlled?

There are a large number of factors that may reduce the accuracy of the BP reading. Your GP may respond appropriately to these seemingly high readings by changing your antihypertensive drugs. The result can be to lower your reading, which is actually within the normal range, thereby predisposing you to dizziness and falls. However, your GP may alternatively discount the readings, assuming they are inaccurate when they are in fact correct – thereby misinterpreting an unacceptably high reading.

> You should always keep your appointments and arrange the next one rather than expect the surgery to send for you

Many people forget to come regularly for their check-ups. Please do not rely on your surgery to call you when your next check-up is due. This is a low priority for surgeries. The time it takes the surgery to recognize that you are overdue for an appointment and then contact you may be time that you have spent with uncontrolled hypertension.

Taking responsibility

It is both important and in your best interest for you to take some responsibility for the management of your hypertension. This should at least include:

❖ coming to your appointments regularly

❖ doing all you can to ensure that the surgery readings are accurate.

> Your doctor may suggest 'self blood pressure measurement' to encourage you to take responsibility for managing your BP

Some people find that they get lower readings when seeing their practice nurse; doing this a couple of times prior to your doctor's appointment can be worthwhile.

However, your GP may think that there are benefits in you taking on more responsibility for your blood pressure management. As mentioned in Chapter 3 (p25), with the advent of accurate automated machines, **self blood pressure measurement** (SBPM) is becoming more accepted by doctors and more popular with the public. This is analogous to:

❖ diabetics checking their own blood sugar levels

❖ asthmatics checking their peak-flow readings.

It is now accepted that increased involvement by the patient in the management of chronic disease pays dividends. Evidence comes from studies of many diseases, such as diabetes and asthma: people do better (in terms of improving their health) and feel more positive if they are involved in the management of their condition. This evidence is still limited for SBPM as accurate automated machines are a recent development. The First International Consensus Conference on Self Blood Pressure Measurement was held as recently as 1999. Until more supportive evidence is available, many doctors will have reasonable concerns about their patients using SBPM.

> Evidence from people with asthma and diabetes suggests that patients tend to feel better and achieve good health faster if they are more heavily involved in the management of their condition

However, the 'partnership' between doctor and patient that can be achieved through SBPM is usually advantageous.

Self blood pressure measurement

This method is not suitable for everyone. Your GP may be concerned about prescribing medication on the basis of readings that cannot be reproduced in the surgery. You may find the prospect of taking your own readings unattractive. However, for the reasons outlined above, it is a step worth seriously considering.

We will go on to describe how you should monitor your BP. However, if you do wish to consider taking this step, it is important to discuss it with the doctor who manages your hypertension.

SBPM machines

You may find it easier and cheaper to get hold of an **aneroid monitor** or non-validated automated monitor. However, your doctor may have reservations about using these readings for continuing management as they are not necessarily reliable. Furthermore, will you have confidence in these readings? One option is to bring your machine in to the surgery and ask your practice nurse to compare your BP readings using the surgery machine and yours.

> Self blood pressure monitors which have an upper arm cuff give the best readings

However, readings can change quite quickly, so this is not ideal. A T-piece can be used to connect both monitors together, but this is time-consuming and complicated and therefore not always popular with the nurse.

The alternative is to buy a machine that you can have more faith in – see Chapter 3 for further details about validated automated monitors. In general, upper arm devices are more accurate than wrist and finger devices.

Taking readings

Chapter 3 discussed in detail how to take a reading. However, from time to time people do encounter difficulties with obtaining a measurement.

One common problem is that the machine produces an error message instead of a BP reading. This kind of unexpected occurrence can cause considerable anxiety, but please don't worry about it – just try again later. If you are getting persistent error messages and yet the machine seems to work on other people, your practice nurse will be able to check your blood pressure and review your technique, so make an appointment and take your machine with you. If you have an irregular pulse, automated monitors may not be suitable for you, as they tend to continually give error messages.

> If you have an irregular pulse, automated machines may not be suitable as they are liable to error

Another difficulty people face is obtaining very variable readings:

* high readings can cause anxiety
* variable readings can cause confusion and ultimately a lack of confidence.

However, changeable readings are a normal occurrence. When starting out, it can be useful to obtain readings at different times of the day. In this way you will get a clearer idea of what your average BP is and the time of day when your reading most closely reflects this. Subsequently, sticking to one time of day will make it easier for you to observe changes in your BP over time.

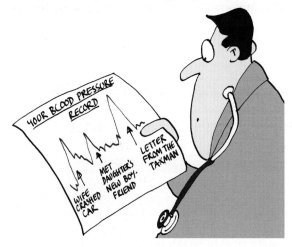

Finally, people commonly find that taking two measurements a few minutes apart results in a lower reading on the second occasion. It is important to repeat the measurement, as it allows time for your blood pressure to settle, as well as allowing the cuff to settle on your arm. Please only record the final reading.

Frequency of measurement

The ideal frequency of measurements is subjective. It is dependent on factors such as:

* how useful to you and your doctor a large number of readings are
* the possible disadvantages associated with becoming obsessed with repeating readings.

Your doctor may have a view on the appropriate frequency of BP measurements in your current situation.

It is common to suggest one reading every two weeks when monitoring a relatively stable blood pressure. This could be increased to weekly measurements when changing treatments. An important medical text on hypertension suggests taking measurements in the morning and evening for one week a quarter when stable, or for one week after changing treatment.

Recording and presentation of readings

You may end up with a number of readings and wish to know the best way to record and submit them to your doctor. You should keep a record of all the readings (exclud-

> It is more useful for your doctor to see the raw data produced by your monitor rather than a chart or graph

ing initial high readings which quickly settled) so that your doctor has the opportunity to review them all. Graphs seem to be popular, but are actually much less useful than the raw data. An average of all readings since your last appointment would also be useful.

How often to see your doctor or nurse

One of the advantages of SBPM is that your GP may be content to see you less regularly. Our practice is to review people with well-controlled blood pressure every six months, but this may vary between doctors.

However, there are some situations in which you may want to go to your surgery early:

❖ It is uncommon for the BP to be so high that it may cause an immediate event, such as a brain haemorrhage. A reading of 220 mmHg systolic or 120 mmHg diastolic that is repeatedly recorded is a cause for concern and probably merits a visit to your doctor that day. This would be an exceptionally rare occurrence.

❖ Much more common is a one-off reading below 220/120 mmHg, but considerably above your usual or target readings. Your GP is unlikely to act on the basis of this one result and there is therefore little point in making an emergency appointment.

> If your home readings are satisfactory, it may only be necessary to see your GP once every six months or so

❖ If your reading is marginally above your usual or target readings, but is lower than 160/100 mmHg, you should continue to take readings as normal and discuss them at your next appointment. If your next appointment is some months away, you may wish to bring it forward; however, readings over the next month or so will help you and your GP decide whether this is a temporary rise, so don't make the appointment too soon.

❖ If your reading is considerably elevated, eg consistently above 160/100 mmHg, it would be sensible to bring the appointment forward. Again, one month's observation prior to the appointment would help your doctor by confirming that this is a persistent change.

How low should the target blood pressure be?

It can be said with reasonable conviction that the lower the BP, the better. The aim must be to achieve the levels indicated in Chapter 4 (page 32). Guidelines for the ideal SBP do vary a little between countries, but a DBP below 90 mmHg seems to be fairly widely agreed. An SBP of 140 or less is regarded as desirable in the American and World Health Organization guidelines. However, the British guidelines suggested a target of 160 mmHg until recently! In this country the figure of 140 has now gained much more widespread acceptance and readers are urged to adopt a level of 140/90 as a maximum and not to be content with anything higher – at least for home readings.

Perhaps achievable targets are 140/85 at home and 150/90 in the surgery. The ideal may be 125/85 in younger age groups and a major study among diabetics in the UK indicated that lives can be saved by aiming for levels of 140/80 or lower.

In people aged over 65 years, such tight control of BP could pose the danger of periodic episodes of significantly lower BP with their associated hazards of fainting and falling.

Achieving your target blood pressure

There are a number of personal factors that may prevent you and your doctor managing your BP effectively. For instance, treating hypertension 'aggressively' (ie trying to rapidly reach your target blood pressure) is often not rewarding to doctors:

❖ The treatment doesn't make you feel better and may in fact make you feel worse. (One of the basic guidelines of medical practice, the Hippocratic oath, commands 'First, do no harm'.) Doctors are well aware that a patient experiencing side-effects to a drug will soon let them know!

❖ You have made it clear to your doctor that you are prepared to try medication. In fact, you have persevered with frequent appointments over a number of months in order to find the treatment that works for you. In this situation, your GP will not want to disappoint you with the bad news that your BP control is still poor. It is therefore important to show your enthusiasm for good BP control.

One other factor that will make reaching your target BP hard is a lack of continuity. Visiting the same physician is recognized as being important for the management of chronic diseases, although seeing your usual doctor may require some forward planning to secure an appointment.

Communicating with your GP

GPs do not always fully explain their actions. Often, this reflects the pressure on their time. However, sometimes it is simply that they are not aware that an explanation is wanted. It is therefore important to ask!

A common example of this is the decision-making process when choosing an antihypertensive drug. GP prescribing is analysed by the Prescribing Pricing Authority (PPA) and the results are made available to GPs and primary care groups (the organizations responsible for an area's drug budget).

> When visiting your GP or practice nurse, take the opportunity to ask questions to help you fully appreciate how to manage your blood pressure

Cost of drugs

There is a common misconception that the cost of prescribed drugs is taken out of a GP's budget. This is not true, and your doctor will not withhold effective drugs from you due to their cost. Each primary care group has an obligation to ensure that it meets its budget and does therefore apply some pressure to GPs. However, this pressure is mainly targeted towards encouraging good medical practice.

Pressure from drug companies

Pharmaceutical companies have a large workforce of sales people dedicated to persuading GPs to prescribe their drug. However, the Department of Health and the General Medical Council now have firm guidelines that strictly limit the hospitality and other benefits that GPs receive from such companies without declaring them.

> When prescribing for hypertension, the majority of GPs in the UK use the guidelines set out by the British Hypertension Society

Guidelines

Up to date information and guidance on good medical practice is more easily available to doctors than ever before. Most British GPs will base prescribing for hypertension on guidelines provided by the British Hypertension Society.

Experience

Personal experience has a major impact on the prescribing habits of doctors. This has definite advantages:

❖ your doctor will have a repertoire of drugs that he or she knows very well

❖ he or she is more likely to be able to predict a drug's effects, including its side-effects

❖ experience may also have convinced him or her to allow new drugs some time to establish a safety record prior to prescribing them.

Being a 'guinea pig'

If your GP or hospital specialist asks if you would be willing to participate in a trial (eg of a new drug or to obtain further information about an existing drug), you may feel inclined to agree for unselfish motives. However, another likely implication is a period of close medical surveillance of your BP.

Summary points

❖ If you are relying on surgery readings, come regularly for your check-ups and try to improve the accuracy of the surgery readings by arriving early, on a day that your are not in a hurry.

❖ There is good evidence that having more involvement in your condition is associated with successful treatment and a greater degree of well being.

❖ If you undertake SBPM, use a machine recommended by the British Hypertension Society.

❖ Keep to the frequency of SBPM readings recommended by your surgery: there will probably be little benefit in doing it more often.

❖ Try not to become anxious over one high reading or an error message.

❖ Be enthusiastic with your treatment, but do ask if you have questions about your hypertension.

Chapter Twelve

Low blood pressure

The lower the blood pressure (BP) the better – or is it? Here we examine the idea that blood pressure can be **too low** and without an identifiable cause. We also look at low blood pressure, or **hypotension**, as a result of drugs or disease and see that it can have sinister connotations. Under these circumstances, low BP can be anything but beneficial and can indeed have some very unpleasant consequences.

Does low blood pressure matter?

They say that when you are choosing an accountant, you should ask all the candidates what two and two make.

♥ The answers three or five are wrong.

♥ The answer four is hopelessly uncreative.

♥ The correct answer is an evasive 'it all depends'!

That is also the answer to the question posed above. Having a 'lowish' blood pressure usually does not matter if it is just an incidental finding during a routine check-up.

> Developing a low blood pressure as a result of taking medication or having a disease can have serious consequences

But if it is the result of medication or of disease, then it does matter, especially if it is low enough to cause adverse symptoms.

Hypotension in the otherwise healthy

In several European countries, especially Germany and France, BPs that we accept as being towards the lower end of the normal range have always been regarded as quite abnormal. People in these countries who have a systolic BP anywhere between 90 and 110 mmHg are thought to suffer from 'low blood pressure'. A very large number of people in these countries are on medication or other therapies to attempt to elevate their BP.

Having a low BP is regarded as providing an explanation for a wide range of extremely prevalent, but non-specific, symptoms. These symptoms include:

❖ lethargy

❖ weakness

❖ fatigue

❖ palpitations

❖ dizziness

❖ faintness.

As long ago as 1940, an American physician pointed out two facts which have since been confirmed. First, that people with low blood pressure tend to live longer than those with a 'normal' BP. Second, that most of the symptoms mentioned above are in fact more common in people with hypertension. Since then, physicians in English-speaking countries have traditionally dismissed so-called **constitutional hypotension** as a spurious condition, and if anything, a rather enviable situation. This subject was re-examined in Australia in 1989 and again in the UK in 1990. Both these studies appeared to demonstrate a relationship between tiredness and low BP, although the results were much more vague regarding the other symptoms considered.

In the UK and the USA it still remains unconventional to offer people medication for low blood pressure.

Hypotension due to medication

There are two rather different situations in which medication can give rise to hypotension:

❖ A drug given for the treatment of hypertension may be prescribed at a dose that is too high, or may simply be too powerful. The hypertension may be much less severe than the doctor thinks, perhaps because he or she has failed to make allowances for the 'white coat' effect (Chapter 3, p26). Some other illness may have intervened to affect the BP – someone taking drugs for hypertension who then suffers a heart attack which can 'magically cure' the hypertension may be unaware of their new lower BP, and may carry on taking the antihypertensive medication.

There are two ways that drugs can cause hypotension:

❖ drugs for hypertension can be prescribed at too high a dose

❖ drugs given for an unrelated condition can lower the blood pressure

❖ Numerous drugs given for totally unrelated conditions can cause hypotension. Such medicines are often given to people with perfectly normal BPs or to people with conditions which can themselves lower the BP. This unwanted BP-lowering effect can present considerable problems in such people. Once again, older people tend to be at greater risk. Some of these drugs are listed in Table 12.1.

Table 12.1 Drugs that may cause hypotension

Class of drug	Example(s)	Condition being treated
ACE inhibitors	Enalapril (Innovace)	Heart failure
Alpha receptor antagonists	Doxazosin, terazosin, indoramin	Enlargement of the prostate
Anaesthetics	Spinal anaesthesia	Surgical procedures (including Caesarean section)
Analgesics	Morphine, diamorphine	Pain, acute heart failure
Antidepressants	Amitriptyline (Tryptizol), other tricyclic compounds	Depression
Beta-blockers	Propranolol (Inderal)	Angina, other heart disorders
Diuretics	Furosemide (Lasix)	Heart failure, fluid retention
Levodopa	Co-careldopa (Sinemet), co-beneldopa (Madopar)	Parkinson's disease
Nitrates	Glyceryl trinitrate, longer-acting nitrates	Angina
Recreational drugs	Cannabis	Causes vasodilatation, hence users get bloodshot eyes
Tranquillizers	Chlorpromazine (Largactil), thioridazine (Melleril), haloperidol (Serenace)	Psychiatric illness, nausea

Hypotension caused by illness or disease

Shock

A low blood pressure is often seen when someone is in **shock** – always a serious situation. Some of the emergencies which bring 'shocked' patients to the Accident and Emergency department are:

> Shock is characterized by low blood pressure

❖ Loss of circulating blood volume due to haemorrhage – will be obvious in someone seriously injured in an accident, or may be less obvious if it is internal. People can bleed internally into the gut, the blood is then:

- vomited up
- passed via the bowel.

Alternatively the blood may flow into tissues or the body cavity, eg from an aortic aneurysm (Chapter 5, p44).

❖ Loss of fluid – for example weeping from inflamed mucous membranes in the bowel. Cholera would be a classic example, although less dramatic illnesses which have a similar effect are seen in the UK.

❖ Badly disrupted circulation – a severe heart attack can seriously affect the heart muscle's ability to pump the blood forwards. Also, a large **pulmonary embolus** (blood clot travelling through the veins to obstruct the pulmonary arteries) can virtually block the circulation. This is the most serious potential danger of a thrombosis in the veins of the lower extremities, and when occurring after a long flight, deep vein thrombosis has earned widespread notoriety as **economy-class syndrome**.

❖ **Anaphylactic shock** is an uncommon but life-threatening allergic reaction to a particular substance (eg peanuts, bee stings). It is characterized by a profound drop in BP and breathing difficulties caused by leakage of fluid out of the circulation and into the tissues. An injection of adrenaline is the first line of treatment.

Many other grave medical and surgical emergencies may cause the victim to become shocked, ranging from ruptured organs in the abdomen to severe bacterial infections and endocrine disturbances.

Chronic hypotension

There are also some illnesses that usually develop much more slowly and are less dramatic in their effects. These are causes of **chronic** hypotension rather than the **acute** emergencies described above.

❖ Many chronic neurological diseases are liable to affect the autonomic nervous system. This may then cause disturbances of the bladder, bowels and sexual function in males, as well as hypotension due to a loss of sympathetic drive. These diseases include:

Causes of chronic hypotension include chronic neurological diseases and severe heart failure

- peripheral neuropathy of unknown cause
- neuropathies associated with diabetes, alcohol, vitamin deficiency and drugs
- Parkinson's disease.

❖ The plasma volume can become depleted due to diabetes, certain kidney diseases and Addison's disease – a fairly rare condition in which the adrenal glands are failing to produce **corticosteroids** (the opposite of Cushing's syndrome, which was mentioned in Chapter 4, p37).

❖ In severe heart failure with a worn-out ventricle, the BP often falls as the power of the pumping action dwindles.

The effects of hypotension

People who have been hypertensive are more susceptible to the symptoms of hypotension than people with a normal BP. This is because the mechanism whereby the blood supply to the brain is preserved at the expense of that to less critical parts of the body (**autoregulation**, Chapter 2, p16) has become impaired. Autoregulation is often less effective in older people, who are commonly more sensitive to the effects of antihypertensive drugs, beta-blockers being the exception.

> 'Postural' or 'orthostatic' hypotension results if the autonomic nervous system/baroceptor reflex fails to work

Although there may be doubt as to whether having a relatively low BP is a good or bad thing, when the BP is lowered by drugs or by disease it can cause very unpleasant symptoms and can be dangerous. Standing up triggers a reflex via the baroceptors and the sympathetic nervous system, which causes the peripheral resistance and heart rate to increase, thereby preventing any significant fall in BP. When the autonomic nervous system is not working properly this reflex will fail. The resulting drop in BP is known as **postural hypotension** or **orthostatic hypotension**. This is usually defined by a drop of over 20 mmHg in the systolic BP or 10 mmHg in the diastolic BP on standing up. Falls of this magnitude don't always cause symptoms and much greater drops are often recorded.

When there is a sudden reduction in the BP, the blood flow to the brain is reduced and brain function is impaired. This is particularly true if cerebral autoregulation is also defective (as is likely in people who are usually hypertensive – see Figure 12.1). The result may be:

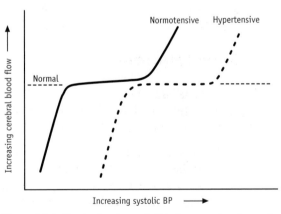

Figure 12.1 Cerebral autoregulation in normotensive and hypertensive individuals. Autoregulation is not as efficient in hypertensive people – it does not start working until the systolic blood pressure is much higher.

> Cerebral blood flow is normally 50–55 mL per 100 g brain per minute; if this falls to 25 mL or less, loss of consciousness may result

❖ loss of consciousness

❖ simply feeling faint

❖ dizziness.

These sensations are very unpleasant and can easily lead to a fall.

For those who like their medical information to be as exact as possible, the cerebral blood flow is normally kept at a remarkably constant 50 to 55 mL per 100 grams of brain per minute, but if this should fall to 25 mL, loss of consciousness may result. A significant fall in cerebral perfusion should not occur until the mean arterial blood pressure drops to around 65 mmHg. Older, frailer people who have weaker bones are more likely to fall and sustain a fracture as a result of having a low BP. Postural hypotension is therefore more dangerous in elderly people but its consequences can affect people of all ages.

Other causes of postural hypotension

Postural hypotension can occur in contexts other than those already mentioned:

❖ Varicose veins are said to predispose to postural hypotension by allowing the blood to pool in the legs.

❖ Prolonged resting can cause reflexes to become dulled by disuse. The most striking example of this results from the weightlessness of space travel, although it is presumed that few of the readers of this book are likely to be astronauts!

❖ There are a few conditions which are increasingly being recognized as causes of suddenly 'coming over faint' – a common scenario, but one which is often difficult to explain. One of the causes is carotid sinus hypersensitivity, in which the baroceptors respond as if the BP was **higher** than it should be so sympathetic drive is reduced which leads to arteriolar dilatation and a slow heartbeat.

❖ Symptoms of hypotension can occur after a large meal, especially if it is largely carbohydrate-based. This is known as **postprandial hypotension** and the drop in BP can occur while the subject is seated at the dining table.

Summary points

❖ Having a slightly lower than normal blood pressure is generally good for the health.

❖ There is some doubt as to whether or not low BP may contribute to a mild sensation of fatigue and possibly other symptoms of a non-specific and not terribly serious nature.

❖ Having a low blood pressure, especially when due to the effects of drugs or neurological disease, can be very unpleasant and lead to faints and falls with potentially serious consequences. Identification of the cause of these conditions can be difficult and treatment is problematic. Any drugs that could cause such problems should be stopped.

❖ A very low blood pressure is also a feature of shock and indicates a life-threatening emergency.

Useful information

The American Heart Association (National Center)
7272 Greenville Avenue
Dallas
TX 75231
USA
Tel: +1 800 242 8751
Web: www.americanheart.org

The American Society of Hypertension
515 Madison Avenue
Suite 1212
New York
NY 10022
USA
Tel: +1 212 644 0650
Fax: +1 212 644 0658
Web: www.ash-us.org

The Blood Pressure Association
60 Cranmer Terrace
London SW17 0AS
UK
Tel: +44 (0)20 8772 4994
Web: www.bpassoc.org.uk

The Blood Pressure Center
HeartCenterOnline
1 South Ocean Boulevard
Suite 301
Boca Raton
FL 33432
USA
Tel: +1 561 620 9790
Web: www.heartcenteronline.com

The British Hypertension Society Information Service
Blood Pressure Unit
Department of Physiological Medicine
St George's Hospital Medical School
Cranmer Terrace
London SW17 0RE
UK
Tel: +44 (0) 20 8725 3412
Web: www.hyp.ac.uk/bhs

European Society for Hypertension
Institute of Clinical & Experimental Medicine
Department of Preventative Cardiology
Videnska 1958/9
140 21 Prague 4
Czech Republic
Web: www.eshonline.org

The High Blood Pressure Foundation
Department of Medical Sciences
Western General Hospital
Edinburgh EH4 2XU
Tel: +44 (0) 131 332 9211
Web: www.hbpf.org.uk

Nurses Hypertension Association
Department of Cardiology
WHRI
University of Wales College of Medicine
Heath Park
Cardiff CF4 4XN
UK
Tel: +44 (0) 29 2074 2352

The World Hypertension League
Tel: +1 800 575 9355
Web: www.mco.edu/org/whl

Websites

www.ash.org.uk	Action on Smoking and Health
www.nutrition.org.uk	British Nutrition Foundation
www.netdoctor.co.uk	An independent health website

Further reading

Beevers DG. *The British Medical Association family doctor guide to blood pressure.* London: Dorling Kindersley 2000.

Beevers DG. *Understanding blood pressure.* London: Family Doctor Publications 2000.

Beevers DG, Lip GYH, O'Brien E. *ABC of hypertension, 4th edn.* London: BMJ Books 2001.

Brewer S. *High blood pressure.* New York: Harper Collins 1997.

Le Fanu J. *The rise and fall of modern medicine.* London: Abacus 1999.

Naqvi NH and Blaufox MD. *Blood pressure measurement: an illustrated history.* New York: Parthenon 1998.

O'Brien E. *Recommendations on blood pressure measurement.* London: BMJ Books 1997.

Pizzarno JE, Murray MT (Eds). *Textbook of natural medicine, 2nd edn.* Edinburgh: Churchill Livingstone 1999.

Shreeve C. *How to lower high blood pressure.* London: Thorsons 2001.

Appendix Two

Coronary risk prediction charts

MEN

SBP = systolic blood pressure (mmHg)
TC:HDL = serum total cholesterol to HDL cholesterol ratio

☐ CHD risk, <15% over next 10 years
▨ CHD risk, 15–30% over next 10 years
■ CHD risk, >30% over next 10 years

CHD risk over next 10 years
15% 20%   30%

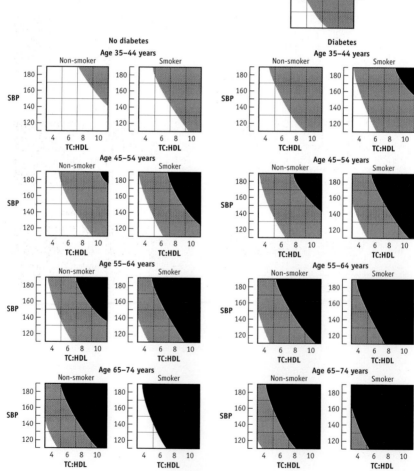

No diabetes

Age 35–44 years

Age 45–54 years

Age 55–64 years

Age 65–74 years

Diabetes

Age 35–44 years

Age 45–54 years

Age 55–64 years

Age 65–74 years

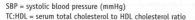

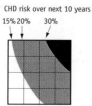

WOMEN

SBP = systolic blood pressure (mmHg)
TC:HDL = serum total cholesterol to HDL cholesterol ratio

☐ CHD risk, <15% over next 10 years
▨ CHD risk, 15–30% over next 10 years
■ CHD risk, >30% over next 10 years

CHD risk over next 10 years
15% 20%   30%

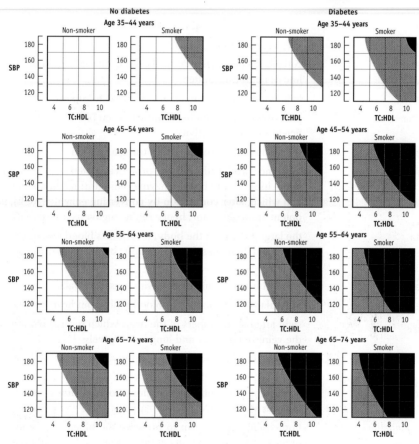

[Reproduced courtesy of Professor Paul Durrington, University of Manchester]

Glossary

acute	very recent onset
adrenergic	connection between nerve cells, using adrenaline or noradrenaline as neurotransmitter
aneurysm	balloon-like swelling in an artery, liable to rupture
angina	pain originating from heart muscle when blood supply is insufficient for current activity
angioplasty	dilatation of a narrowed artery using a balloon
angiotensin	substance produced when the protein angiotensinogen (formed in the liver) is split by the enzyme renin (formed in the kidney) and which, after conversion by converting enzyme (ACE), is a potent vasoconstrictor; hence renin–angiotensin system (RAS)
aorta	the largest artery in the body; it conducts blood away from the heart and branches from it supply blood to the organs and extremities
arteriole	smallest branches of arteries, with muscular walls
artery	muscular vessel conducting blood away from heart
atria	right and left; chambers of the heart which receive blood from the veins of the body and lungs respectively
auscultation	listening to heart, lungs or other organs through a stethoscope, usually done by a health professional
autonomic	acting independently of conscious control, hence autonomic nervous system (ANS)
autoregulation	homeostatic mechanism to preserve the blood supply to vital organs, eg brain, generally at the expense of less vital organs
baroceptors	pressure-sensitive organs
biofeedback training	technique whereby result from a physiological test is relayed directly back to the individual on whom the measurement was made in order to train the subject in taking control of the function being measured
brachial	relating to the arm; brachial artery – main artery supplying blood to the upper limb, easily accessible at bend of elbow
capillaries	smallest branches of circulation, in intimate contact with tissues

capillary bed	sum total of all the capillaries
cardiac	relating to the heart
cardiac output (CO)	quantity of blood pumped from the heart in one minute
cardiovascular	relating to the heart and blood vessels (mainly arteries) – hence cardiovascular system (CVS)
carotid	arteries branching off the aorta to supply the head and brain
cerebral	relating to the brain
cerebrovascular	relating to blood vessels of brain
cholesterol	fatty substance in blood
chronic	long-term, eg chronic illness
coronary	artery supplying blood to heart muscle, hence coronary heart disease (CHD)
corticosteroids	drugs resembling hydrocortisone – a hormone produced by the adrenal glands
diastole	phase of relaxation of ventricles; adj. diastolic
diuretic	effect of causing kidney to produce greater quantities of urine
echocardiogram	examination of heart structure using ultrasound
endothelial cells	cells lining the inside of blood vessels
free radical	a molecule or atom with an unpaired electron – a number of harmful oxygen metabolites are free radicals
gangrene	death of part of the body, usually foot and/or leg, due to loss of blood supply
haemorrhage	to bleed
hemiplegia	paralysis of one side of the body, usually due to stroke
homeostasis	mechanisms for preserving constant internal environment of the body
hormone	chemicals released by glands which exert their effect in distant part of the body from site of release; hence antidiuretic hormone (ADH) reduces urine production, hormone replacement therapy (HRT) for women whose ovaries no longer produce the female sex hormones oestrogen and progesterone
hyper-	prefix indicating too high, too much, hence hypertension
hypertrophy	enlargement of organ due to excessive work, eg left ventricle hypertrophy
hypo-	prefix indicating too low, too little, hence hypotension
infarction	death of tissue
ischaemia	starvation of blood supply to an organ
lumbar	relating to lower spine
lumen	interior of tubular structure
mean arterial pressure (MABP)	diastolic BP plus one-third of pulse pressure

mL	millilitre, a measurement of liquid, a cubic centimetre, one thousandth of a litre
mmHg	millimetres of mercury; standard unit of measurement of blood pressure
myocardial	relating to heart muscle, hence myocardial infarction (MI)
nephritis	inflammation of kidney; pyelonephritis – due to bacterial infection, glomerulonephritis – due to immune mechanism
neurone	nerve cell, part of the central nervous system (CNS)
neurotransmitter	chemical substance which transmits a nervous impulse from one nerve cell to another, or from one nerve cell to an effector cell, eg muscle or gland
oedema	swelling due to fluid accumulation, usually in feet and lower part of legs
ophthalmoscope	instrument for examining blood vessels and other structures within eyeball
osmolality	concentration of solutes in fluid
parasympathetic	part of autonomic nervous system emerging from brain stem and lower part of spinal cord, generally utilizing acetylcholine as the neurotransmitter
perfusion	blood supply of a region or organ
peripheral resistance (PR)	resistance to passage of blood through the smaller vessels of the circulation
polycystic disease	inherited disorder of kidney causing hypertension
pulse pressure	difference between diastolic BP and systolic BP
receptor	part of a cell that receives neurotransmitter so that the cell responds to the impulse
reflex	nervous circuit which bypasses brain and allows a rapid response to an external stimulus
relative risk (RR)	the number of times more likely an event is to happen in one group compared to another – a relative risk less than 1 means that the event is less likely to happen than in the general population
renal	relating to the kidneys
smooth muscle	muscle controlling tubular structures which is in turn controlled by the autonomic nervous system rather than conscious effort
sphygmomanometer	instrument for measuring blood pressure
stenosis	narrowing, eg renal artery stenosis
stroke	damage to part of the brain caused by interruption of blood supply
stroke volume (SV)	quantity of blood pumped out by the heart in to the aorta each time it beats
sympathetic	part of the autonomic nervous system emerging from central parts of spinal cord, generally utilizing adrenaline and noradrenaline as the neurotransmitters

synapse	connection between two neurones
systole	contraction of ventricles; adj. systolic
thoracic	relating to chest or lungs
toxaemia	dangerous condition causing hypertension during pregnancy
vascular	relating to blood vessels
vasoconstriction	action whereby vessels, arterioles in particular, contract and become narrower
vasodilatation	action whereby vessels, arterioles in particular, relax and become wider
vein	vessel carrying blood back towards the heart
ventricles	right and left; muscular chambers of the heart which receive blood from the atria and eject it into the lungs and aorta respectively
venules	capillaries rejoin each other to form these smallest constituents of the venous circulation

Index

Note: Page numbers in *italics* represent figures and tables.

Since the major subject of this book is blood pressure, entries have been kept to a minimum under this term and readers are advised to seek more specific index entries.

Abbreviations used in this index include:

ACE – angiotensin-converting enzyme
BP – blood pressure
CHD – coronary heart disease
DBP – diastolic blood pressure
SBP – systolic blood pressure

N

O

P

X

Z

Y